PCOS

D1044034

PCOS

A WOMAN'S GUIDE TO DEALING WITH POLYCYSTIC OVARY SYNDROME

Colette Harris with Dr Adam Carey

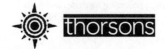

While the authors of this work have made every effort to ensure that the information contained in this book is as accurate and up to date as possible at the time of publication, medical and pharmaceutical knowledge is constantly changing and the application of it to particular circumstances depends on many factors. Therefore it is recommended that readers always consult a qualified medical specialist for individual advice. This book should not be used as an alternative to seeking specialist medical advice, which should be sought before any action is taken. The authors and publishers cannot be held responsible for any errors and omissions that may be found in the text, or any actions that may be taken by a reader as a result of any reliance on the information contained in the text, which is taken entirely at the reader's own risk.

Thorsons
An Imprint of HarperCollins*Publishers*
77–85 Fulham Palace Road,
Hammersmith, London W6 8JB

The website address is: www.thorsonselement.com

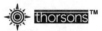

and *Thorsons* are trademarks of
HarperCollins*Publishers* Limited

Published by Thorsons 2000

15 17 19 20 18 16 14

© Colette Harris and Dr Adam Carey 2000

Colette Harris and Dr Adam Carey assert the
moral right to be identified as the authors of this work

A catalogue record for this book
is available from the British Library

ISBN 0 7225 3975 4

Printed and bound in Great Britain by
Martins The Printers Ltd, Berwick upon Tweed

All rights reserved. No part of this publication may be
reproduced, stored in a retrieval system, or transmitted,
in any form or by any means, electronic, mechanical,
photocopying, recording or otherwise, without the prior
permission of the publishers.

For women with PCOS and the people who support them.

Contents

Acknowledgements

Colette:

A huge thank-you to Chris, my partner, for his faith in me and encouragement, to my wonderful family and friends for their support, to my work colleagues for lending a sympathetic ear, to Verity – especially Jacqui and Una – for all they are doing to raise awareness of PCOS, to Victoria at Thorsons for believing in the project and helping it come to light, and to Adam for giving the benefit of his scientific knowledge to this book.

Adam:

I would like to thank my wife Beverly and my son Matthew and the rest of our family for their continuing help and support whilst writing this. I know it was not easy but it needed doing. Thanks to my friends and colleagues for putting up with me, and especially thanks to Colette without whom this book would not have occurred.

Foreword

The polycystic ovary syndrome (PCOS) is the commonest hormonal disturbance to affect women. Approximately one fifth of women have polycystic ovaries and maybe a half to three-quarters of these experience symptoms at some time in their lives. Symptoms can include: irregular periods, unwanted bodily hair or acne and problems with being overweight. There may also be some longer term risks to health, such as an increased risk of developing diabetes and heart disease.

In recent times we have learnt more about the causes of PCOS and the situations which can make the symptoms better – or worse. There now exist a number of medical treatments for the management of associated menstrual irregularity, infertility and unwanted hair growth/acne. It is important, however, to take an holistic approach and consider appropriate diets, exercise and ways of reducing stress. Colette Harris provides in this book a comprehensive account of PCOS and how to manage the many varied aspects of this complex condition. Colette talks with authority having undertaken considerable research in the area and is to be congratulated on her pragmatic approach, which I am sure will be of benefit to all of those who read it.

Adam H. Balen MD, MRCOG
Consultant Obstetrician and Gynaecologist
Subspecialist in Reproductive Medicine, Leeds General Infirmary

Introduction

Despite being a health journalist, when I was finally diagnosed with PCOS in December 1996 I was none the wiser. What on earth was 'polycystic ovary syndrome'? If I had never heard of it, and my doctor said there was no cure, then surely that meant it was rare and I would never get any better.

The only clue I had about what the lumpy spots, fatigue, joint pain, hair loss, lack of periods and sudden boom in weight actually meant was the 'reassurance' I was given by the technician who had taken my ultrasound scan. 'Don't worry,' he had said, 'there's a lot they can do to help women who can't have children nowadays. Don't you go getting yourself upset.'

What else did he expect me to do? After eight months of failing health, and despair about ever getting my doctor to take me seriously, I had my diagnosis at last. It shed no light on anything, apart from leaving me with the fear that I would never be able to have children without medical intervention.

I was glad I had a name for my hideous collection of symptoms, glad that I could tell people I'd 'got' something so they wouldn't think I was malingering or trying to skip work and seeing family and friends because I simply couldn't be bothered. But saying I had PCOS meant nothing to anyone, least of all me.

The fact that various doctors in the collective practice I was then registered with knew little or nothing about it either, didn't help. I was bewildered, frightened because I was told there was 'no cure' and left with my self-esteem in shreds. I didn't want to be fat and spotty, be so tired that I could sleep for 17 hours on a Friday night and be ready for bed again only four hours after I woke up. And I didn't want to feel unfeminine, with darkening hairs on my upper lip and a sense that my body might not be able to produce children should I decide that would be a good idea. However limiting that definition of femininity is, I would be lying if I said those things didn't affect me. I was tired, moody, resentful that my doctor couldn't tell me more about what was going on inside my body, in a constant state of PMS muddled-headedness and I felt hopelessly unattractive.

I was told there was nothing I could do except go on the Pill. I didn't want to. I had taken it before and always felt not quite right. I had put on weight, had constant dizzy spells and fainted fairly regularly while I was taking a variety of different brands one after another. So I asked about my other options and was told there weren't any. I pushed for a referral to a specialist. The nearest I could get was for April the following year. So I had four and half months to either put up with my symptoms or become a PCOS detective. I chose not to put up with illness any longer.

As luck would have it, the December issue of the magazine I work on, *Here's Health*, had a story in it about a woman with multiple cysts on her ovaries who had found it difficult to conceive. She had received herbal treatments which had restored her periods. I wondered if her multiple cysts were in fact a sign of PCOS. I pestered my doctor, who managed to find me a leaflet.

PCOS stands for polycystic ovary *syndrome*, which is the name given to the condition which includes having polycystic ovaries (PCO) *and* symptoms associated with the syndrome – you can have PCO without having PCOS, which is why the two are sometimes referred to jointly as PCO/S.

The leaflet my doctor gave me on PCO/S was surprisingly informative and helped me to understand the basics as they then stood. (Research has since found many more interesting explanations of how PCO/S works and develops, which you will find throughout this book.) I grasped that PCO/S was about a hormonal imbalance, with too much oestrogen and increased testosterone in the blood and not enough follicle stimulating hormone (FSH) in the ovaries to release an egg regularly. I was privileged to have access to a mine of information on alternative health and nutrition from the *Here's Health* library, and slowly but surely, after talking to herbalists and nutritional therapists and reading several books and health encyclopaedias, I began to try out a fairly drastic health regime. The basics were a wholefood vegan diet with no alcohol or caffeine, herbal and nutritional supplements, filtered water and gentle exercise.

My periods, which had finally disappeared completely in August 1996, four months before my diagnosis, came back within the month. Weight started to come off, my painful acne-type spots receded, my hair stopped falling out and my moods began to level off.

It was just after New Year when good luck stepped in and I got a call from Jacqui Garnier at the office. Jacqui was a member of a fledgling organization called Verity, whose aim was to become a self-help group for women with PCOS. She was asking if our magazine could run features on it. We got talking and I realized that there were a lot of women like me out there, wondering what they could do to understand their condition and help themselves.

In April the consultant gynaecologist I had waited so long to see told me that the improvements in my health were beyond anything she'd usually seen with the prescriptions she recommended to women under her care. I was told I might as well carry on doing what I was doing. While in one way this made me feel great, because it vindicated my dietary approach to managing PCO/S, I was also very disappointed that I hadn't been given more options to explore. It seemed that the health professionals I had come across knew little about PCOS and didn't really seem to understand how much it affects the lives of women who have it. I felt angry that I hadn't had the confidence to say so in my consultation.

By July 1997 I was pretty much well again. My periods were regular as clockwork and my life was on a much more even keel, as were my moods and my hormones. I still got (and do get) PMS symptoms for a week before my period, to a varying degree of severity depending on how stressed I've been in the month beforehand. But six or seven days of tender breasts and irritability is such an improvement in my health that I practically welcome them every month, knowing as I do now that there will be a period at the end of it.

My symptoms do creep back in on me if I eat unhealthily for a month. So there's no denying that it can be hard work and that sometimes I just have to be kind to myself – if I start daydreaming about chocolate or some chips then I just have some and let it go. But the longer I do without, the less intense I find the cravings are – now they're linked more to stress and an emotional link to comfort eating than to PMS.

I felt I should write about what had happened to me so that women without access to the information I had could realize there were other ways to help deal with PCO/S and that they weren't on their own, even though it was a bit embarrassing for me to talk about having excess hair on my lip, and quite hard to persuade people that PCOS was a condition worth writing about. The response to articles in newspapers and magazines was astonishing. It seemed many women with PCO/S felt too scared to talk about it – the stigma attached to infertility and symptoms such as body hair had kept it hidden, even among the often emotionally honest conversations of women with other women. What was also interesting was that several women wrote letters to me saying that they had been dealing with the type of symptoms mentioned in the articles without going to the doctor because they had just assumed they were unlucky with their skin or their weight. Having read the articles, they were going to get appointments with their doctors to see if they had PCO/S.

With Verity's details at the end of the articles, lots of women finally got to make contact with other women who felt like they did. PCO/S was finally coming out of the woodwork, but it still has a long way to go in order to become more readily recognized.

The aim of this book, which I have written along with Dr Adam Carey, is to reach even more women who have PCOS or who are experiencing strange symptoms that could be PMS but somehow feel more than that. In a way I hope it is slightly out of date by the time you read it – that would mean more research has been done on the condition. Chances are it's bang up to date, but we can hope!

We aim to raise awareness and give practical support. Ideally we would like the book to help prevent any more women experiencing such a sense of fear and helplessness when diagnosed with PCOS. The book is designed to be an empowering source of both information and strategies for self-help, born from a rare collaboration between a patient and a health professional, both of whom feel that women with PCOS – and those who support them – deserve a better deal.

We don't claim to have all the answers. But we do know that PCOS need not be a life sentence of ill-health, struggle, despair and low self-esteem. As someone once said, knowledge is power. We hope the knowledge you gain from these pages will help you feel ready to take charge of your health, be more confident in your relationship with your doctor and more accepting and loving towards your body. As someone else once said, no one said it would be easy. But we hope this book and the useful organizations listed at the end can make it a whole lot easier than it used to be.

PCOS? Never heard of it!

'Why have I never heard of PCOS?' Many women ask this question when they are diagnosed, or are asked it when they try and explain to someone what's been making them feel under the weather. It is amazing that a condition estimated by the medical profession to affect up to one in ten women can be so unheard of.

THE HUSH HUSH FACTOR

The main problem for women with PCO/S, aside from the ill-health, is that their condition is so little known or talked about that it leaves them feeling isolated and powerless.

Few women know about PCOS until they are diagnosed with it. Everyone who has felt their chest go suddenly tight and wheezy might wonder whether they have developed asthma; most women who feel a burning sensation when they pee would suspect that perhaps they have cystitis. But many women who have any number of symptoms associated with PCOS might not be able to guess at it nor ask their doctor to rule it out, because it's still a hush hush condition.

PCOS OR PMS?

It might seem surprising to have to look back as far as the 1930s, but a brief dip into history can tell us a lot. In the 1930s – when PCOS was first 'discovered' and named by two doctors called Stein and Leventhal – only women who were very overweight, had no periods at all and also showed a lot of facial or body hair were classed as having PCOS.

Very little research was carried out for the following 60 years, so many women dealing with the day-to-day problems that PCOS can bring – in whatever shape, form or severity – would not have been classified as having the condition.

Even now, the three symptoms mentioned above – overweight, no periods at all and an overgrowth of facial or body hair – are considered to be the 'classic' signs of PCOS that healthcare practitioners look out for. Yet there is a whole menu of symptoms associated with PCOS, including the three mentioned above but also covering such experiences as fatigue, acne, joint pain, hair loss (alopecia), tender breasts, bloating, mood swings, difficulty in conceiving and depression. A woman with PCOS could display any single one or any combination of these symptoms, which can make it very difficult to diagnose.

Helen, 28, for example, only ever had acne and depression, so was given antibiotics, told she was stressed out, and then referred to a counsellor for her depression:

❋ *The way my symptoms were looked at separately by my doctor meant that I never connected them together either. It was my mum who said that she sometimes got depressed before a period – that got me wondering. I realized I'd always had a really long cycle of around 38 days, but had never told my doctor because it had always been like that. When I did tell him he started to think around the acne, blue moods and irregular periods, and diagnosed PCOS.*

On the other hand, Amber, now 35, never had any symptoms to speak of but just found it hard to get pregnant:

We tried for four years before we managed to have Thomas with IVF treatment. It was only during a scan during the treatment that someone pointed out that I have PCOS. Had I known about it four years before, we could have saved a lot of heartache.

One in five women who has ultrasound scans during gynaecological examinations show up polycystic ovaries.[1] Of those who are found to have polycystic ovaries on ultrasound scan, more than 80 per cent do in fact have one or more of the classic symptoms of PCOS, although they have not complained of these symptoms.[2] These women considered themselves normal and had not complained before the ultrasound examination questionnaire.

PCOS is polycystic ovary syndrome, which is the name given to the condition which includes having polycystic ovaries *and* symptoms associated with the syndrome – you can have PCO without having PCOS.

FACT: PERIODS ARE A PROBLEM

It is also worth noting that many women are brought up to think that periods are a 'curse' and bring pain, acne and bad moods with them as a matter of course. If you are brought up to expect pain and misery as normal, you won't go to see a doctor to check if there's anything wrong if you experience them. Women who have scanty, light or even non-existent periods often feel they are getting off lightly and shouldn't complain. Many women with PCOS who have this problem have in fact been told that they are 'lucky' by doctors.

If more women felt they had a right to expect more regular – in both senses of the word – periods, more women would go to the doctor and insist that they be checked out for gynaecological problems such as PCOS.

STRESSED OUT?

There is a danger that because stress is known to have such wide-ranging effects in people – from heart attacks and stomach ulcers to fatigue and insomnia – it can almost be blamed for anything, including the sorts of symptoms associated with PCO/S. Acne, weight gain, fatigue, hair loss, even irregular periods can all so easily be attributed to stress that the comfort of self-diagnosing ourselves and recommending to ourselves that we take it easier can leave the PCOS stone unturned.

TOO GUILTY TO PAY ATTENTION TO OURSELVES?

It is still a commonly held belief that women are supposed to sacrifice everything to help others, because women are supposed to have the 'mothering instinct'. This can leave women who worry about their own health feeling guilty. How many of us brush aside worries because we feel we don't want to cause a fuss?

AN EMBARRASSING TOPIC

PCOS can be hard to talk about because it deals with embarrassing and emotionally-charged topics such as excess body hair, adult acne, periods and fertility issues. And let's face it, talking to friends about these things can be hard enough, never mind a doctor, especially when you are feeling low. But talking about these sorts of problems is the first step to getting the right kind of help.

THE FEAR THAT COMES WITH CHANGE

Feelings of bewilderment, and shame about the changes that can happen in a woman's body and emotional life if she has PCOS, can be very frightening.

❋ *These mood swings took over my life. I would be really snappy one minute, weepy the next and then laugh at things that weren't really funny at all. I felt out of control. Emma, 24*

❋ *I was disgusted by how my body started to look. I sprouted hair round my nipples, navel, and on my chin. I refused to look in the mirror unless I was shaving it off. I was too ashamed to see a beautician. I thought I was turning into a man because of the hair and because my waist disappeared under the extra pounds that piled on. I was a nervous wreck by the time I was desperate enough to see a doctor. Sheila, 36*

DOCTOR, DOCTOR

If you feel as demoralized, upset and frightened as Emma and Sheila did by the time you get to the doctor, it can be easy to let them tell you there's nothing really wrong, that many women have body hair, that many women feel tired, moody and put on weight as they get older. This is partly because when you're feeling down and at a low ebb anyway it's very hard to stand up for yourself against a trained professional who feels there is little worth investigating. We are also taught from an early age to trust what doctors tell us – but bear in mind that PCOS is a condition still very much in the shadows, so it could be simply that your doctor doesn't know very much about it. (If you think this is the case, ask them directly if they think it could be PCOS.) It can also be easy to accept a pat answer because, despite knowing deep down that there is something wrong, you want to hear that there is not.

IT'S GOOD TO TALK

In the end it's down to us to take responsibility for our own health when we can. If we talk to our friends, doctors, families and other women with

PCOS we can help to shed light on what it is and help to determine the right way for it to be treated.

The more information we share about PCOS and our feelings about dealing with it, the less it will remain ignored and under-recognized.

What Is Polycystic Ovary Syndrome?

Polycystic ovary syndrome is a health condition linked with hormonal imbalances and insulin resistance, which can bring about a whole menu of symptoms, from irregular or non-existent periods to excess body hair, acne and weight gain along with fatigue, depression, acne, hair loss and other less common symptoms (see list on page 14).

It is estimated that one in ten women has this condition, even though many of them may not know it because their symptoms may be diagnosed as PMS, for example.

The basic cause of PCOS is believed to involve an inability of the ovaries to produce hormones in the correct proportions. The pituitary gland senses that the ovary is not working properly, and in turn releases abnormal amounts of luteinizing hormone (LH) and follicle stimulating hormone (FSH), which are both linked to the ovary's ability to develop and release an egg. It is when this ability to ovulate becomes disabled that infertility can occur in women with PCOS.

Irving Stein and Michael Leventhal first described the condition in 1934.[1] In order to name this 'new' disorder they used the example of seven women who could not fall pregnant, who were overweight, had excess body and facial hair and whose ovaries showed up lots of tiny cysts on

X-ray. Because techniques for diagnosing health conditions were less advanced then, only women with these symptoms at an extreme stage were labelled as having PCOS. In reality, you can have PCOS even if you don't have all these 'classic' symptoms.

Not every woman with PCOS suffers with all the related symptoms. You can have any combination of them to any degree of severity, or even have no obvious symptoms at all except the cysts on your ovaries that give the condition its name.

WHAT DO POLYCYSTIC OVARIES LOOK LIKE?

'Polycystic' literally means 'many cysts'. Polycystic ovaries have a string of cysts around their outside. There are usually around ten or more, which can be described as a 'pearl necklace' effect. The cysts are small, usually measuring 2 to 8 millimetres across. Figure 1 below illustrates a normal ovary; Figure 2 a polycystic ovary.

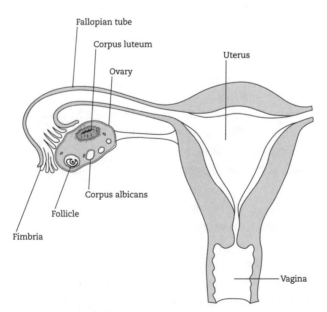

Figure 1: A normal ovary

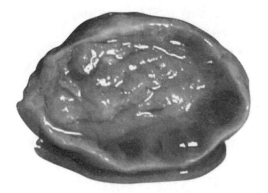

Figure 2: A polycystic ovary

When the ovary is viewed using an ultrasound scan, the same features can be clearly seen (Figure 3). Having at least 10 cysts with thickened stroma which appear brighter than normal (stroma is the name given to the tissue within the ovary that is not the follicles, made of thecal cells) on the scan enables a diagnosis of polycystic ovaries.[2,3,4]

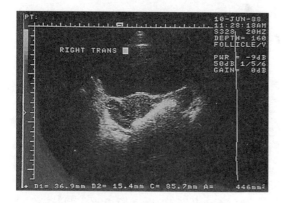

Figure 3

SO ARE THE CYSTS THE PROBLEM?

Many people wonder if the cysts are the problem, and ask if the symptoms of PCOS would go away if the cysts were removed. However, the cysts are actually a *symptom* of the condition, not its cause. They are different to ovarian cysts, which are usually single and can grow bigger and interfere with the function of the ovary. In PCOS the string of small cysts seen in the outer edge of the ovary are thought to be follicles that have failed to develop completely to release an egg. There can be a hormonal imbalance which encourages the ovaries to produce follicles to house developing eggs, but doesn't produce the right amount of other hormones needed to stimulate the egg to mature. So you can get empty follicles which show up as dark blobs on the ultrasound and are called cysts. They are actually a consequence of the hormonal malfunction in a woman with PCOS rather than the cause of it.

CAN YOU HAVE THE CYSTS BUT NOT THE SYNDROME?

Women with polycystic ovaries and one or more of the classic symptoms are said to have polycystic ovary syndrome (PCOS). But not all women with polycystic ovaries on an ultrasound scan (PCO) would end up with symptoms, so they would not be described as having the syndrome.

Many women who are shown to have polycystic ovaries on an ultrasound scan don't actually have any of the symptoms of the syndrome. So 'normal' women can have polycystic ovaries.

When a woman is symptom-free, the polycystic ovaries show that she has an in-built predisposition to developing PCOS. If she puts on weight or comes under a great deal of stress she may develop the symptoms.

Finding the polycystic ovaries, therefore, can be a useful way to warn someone that she should look after herself to make sure she doesn't develop PCOS in the future.

CAN THE CYSTS BE REMOVED?

The cysts seen in PCOS are symptoms of the deeper underlying hormonal and metabolic problems which cause the syndrome. If you get these underlying problems sorted out, or improved, the cysts will often disappear or reduce in number.

Trying to remove the cysts surgically would mean removing a large amount of the ovary itself. If too much of the ovary is lost there will be no further eggs left to develop each month and the ovaries will stop functioning. When the ovaries stop functioning a woman's periods will stop completely and she will commonly experience menopausal symptoms such as night sweats.

Premature menopause or ovarian failure, before the age of 45 years, is highly undesirable because it brings with it associated symptoms and risks such as osteoporosis.

There is a surgical treatment known as ovarian drilling which can help some women with PCOS who don't ovulate and therefore can't get pregnant. This treatment 'jump-starts' the ovaries into releasing some eggs. However it is only a short-term measure which helps for around six months to a year, and can damage the ovary. There are many other, less drastic ways, to help women with PCOS, as will be explored later in this book.

CAN PCOS BE CURED?

The symptoms associated with PCOS, outlined above, are all commonly associated with times of hormonal disturbance such as puberty, pregnancy and menopause. This has led to PCOS being generally classified as a gynaecological disorder, the sort of thing you would sometimes hear described as 'women's troubles'. Taking the contraceptive pill can help to even out the menstrual cycle of a woman with PCOS and mask the symptoms which she can suffer from.

However, research done into PCOS has shown that women with the syndrome are at an increased risk of recurrent miscarriage and developing diabetes and heart disease. It seems that the hormonal symptoms are actually triggered off by a deeper, underlying cause which has long-term health consequences beyond the reproductive lifetime of a woman's body.

The cysts and other symptoms of PCOS develop as a result of a genetic disposition towards PCOS, handed down through the family, as well as environmental factors such as diet, lifestyle and stress levels.

Therefore, although there is no 'cure' for PCOS, and you can do nothing about your inherited genetic make-up, you can deal with the condition and help yourself to feel better by getting to grips with lifestyle changes. There are also many treatments which target specific symptoms such as acne or excess hair.

THE SYMPTOMS OF PCOS

The Classic Symptoms of PCOS

- ✸ irregular periods
- ✸ excessive facial or body hair
- ✸ acne
- ✸ infertility

A number of groups have looked at the incidence of symptoms which patients present with to their doctor. The list below contains data from one such study[5] of 300 women presenting with an ultrasound diagnosis of polycystic ovaries. It is similar to the findings from many other researchers who have reported their findings and where the diagnosis has either been made from either histological sections taken from the ovary as done by Stein and Leventhal or by ultrasound.[6,7]

Symptom	Percentage of women presenting
Irregular cycle (Oligomenorrhoea)	52%
No periods (Amenorrhoea)	28%
Irregular spotting	14%
Extra facial or body hair (Hirsutism)	64%
Acne	27%
Obesity	35%
Infertility	52%

We will now look in more detail at each of the common symptoms of PCOS.

Irregular Periods
These are defined as a menstrual cycle length of less than 21 days or greater than 35 days, or with more than 4 days of variation from month to month. The menstrual period may be consistently irregular with long gaps – known as oligomenorrhoea – or non-existent – known as amenorrhoea. This may result in either irregular ovulation or no ovulation (known as anovulation).

Hirsutism
This is defined as excessive facial or body hair, commonly with a male pattern of distribution.

Acne
This is typically on the face, but can also affect the chest, shoulders and back.

Infertility
This is defined as a failure to conceive after one year of regular unprotected sexual intercourse. Irregular ovulation usually means that pregnancy is more difficult to achieve. If ovulation is not taking place it is not possible to conceive without help.

Obesity

This is normally defined using a weight-to-height ratio. This is called the body mass index (BMI) and is calculated by dividing your weight in kilograms by your height in metres squared. A normal BMI is between 20 and 25.

Other Common Symptoms

Male-pattern Hair Loss

This commonly occurs as thinning from the top of the head or crown, together with loss from the front and a receding hair line.

Miscarriage

This is the loss of a pregnancy in the early part of the development, normally before 14 weeks. Women with PCOS who have high levels of Luteinizing Hormone may be at greater risk of early pregnancy loss.

Pelvic Pain

Some women notice pelvic pain. This may be related to the effect of hormones on the blood flow through the veins within the pelvis.

Other PCOS symptoms include:

- ✿ mood swings
- ✿ breast pain
- ✿ abdominal pain
- ✿ aching joints
- ✿ dizziness
- ✿ increased tendency to faint
- ✿ chronic fatigue.

YOUR QUESTIONS ANSWERED

Do the cysts mean I have ovarian cancer?

The small cysts of PCOS do not need removal and are not a sign of ovarian cancer. However, as with women with a normal ovarian structure, women with PCOS may very rarely get a larger cyst, over 50 millimetres, which will require surgical removal. But women with PCOS are no more or less likely to suffer such a problem than other women, and there is no link between the cysts of polycystic ovaries and ovarian cancer.

Will PCOS go away at menopause when my ovaries stop functioning?
A recent study suggests that many women with PCOS notice that their PCOS symptoms subside somewhat at the time of menopause. However, a small minority of women notice an increase in excess hair after menopause due to abnormal function in their ovaries.

How the Ovary Works

As has been explained earlier, PCOS is a condition linked to hormonal imbalances and other factors such as genetic inheritance and insulin resistance. It is a complicated condition, and in order to help us work out what is going on we need to look at the normal ovary and what it does during the menstrual cycle.

WHERE ARE THE OVARIES?

A woman has two ovaries that lie within the pelvis suspended behind the uterus and Fallopian tubes (see Figure 4). The adult ovary is about the size of a walnut and has a mother of pearl sheen to it.

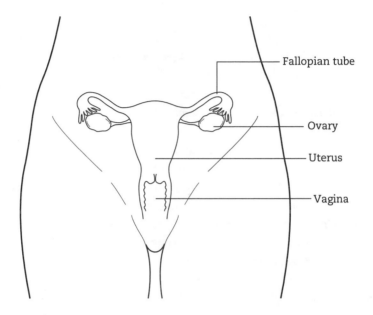

Fallopian tube

Ovary

Uterus

Vagina

Figure 4

Storing Your Eggs

Your store of eggs is allotted to you when you are just a foetus in your own mother's womb.

All eggs initially contain 46 chromosomes, a complete copy of a woman's genetic material, as in all other human cells. But the eggs must undergo a unique cell-division process where the chromosome number is halved in preparation for later fertilization. The number of chromosomes within the egg will be halved from 46 to 23 (22 chromosomes plus the X-chromosome) at the time of the formation of the egg. If fertilized, these 23 chromosomes will be joined by 23 from the sperm (22 plus either the X-chromosome or the Y-chromosome).

Getting to Grips with Our Genes

The whole point of the egg within the ovary is to bring its share of genetic information to the growing foetus, in order to pass on the mother's inherited physical and emotional characteristics. As genetics and inherited health conditions all play a vital role in understanding PCOS, it is useful to pause here and take on board some details about our genes.

All cells within our bodies – with the exception of the developed eggs or sperm – contain 46 chromosomes. Each cell contains 22 pairs of chromosomes and two sex chromosomes. The chromosomes are made from long lengths of DNA (Deoxyribonucleaic acid). The DNA contains the genetic blueprint of life. The two sex chromosomes are either XX for a girl or XY for a boy. It is the genes present on the Y-chromosome that determine that a person is to be male.

The egg and the sperm each only contain 23 chromosomes. The role of the egg is to carry a single copy of the mother's genes (23 chromosomes) on to the next generation. At the time of fertilization the egg and the sperm each bring together half of the genetic material required to form the new embryo. The newly formed embryo has 46 chromosomes.

The reduction in the number of chromosomes in the eggs and the division process is called *meiosis*. All the eggs are left in this state of suspended animation until they are re-awakened one by one after puberty, when the half-developed eggs are stimulated to maturity by the monthly surge of hormones.

Some of the eggs in their primary follicles may stay unawakened for more than 50 years because, unlike men who can produce new sperm cells throughout their lives, women cannot produce new egg cells – they can only develop the ones they were born with. These cells stored in waiting and the genetic material they carry are vulnerable to damage, and this may well explain why there is an increasing incidence of chromosomal malformations such as Down's Syndrome in the children of older women.

Preparing the Eggs for Fertilization

Before puberty is reached, then, each egg in the ovary lies dormant, surrounded by a number of cells which can develop into a follicle – a fluid-filled space that can nurture the egg into a mature egg ripe for fertilization.

In order that an egg can mature and be released each month, a normal menstrual cycle needs to take place. The creation and regulation of this cycle is the job of the ovary itself. The ovary also produces the hormones that co-ordinate the body to be receptive to the fertilized egg.

This co-ordinated control of the follicle growth, the release of the egg and the anticipation of fertilization form the basis of the female menstrual cycle. In order for a woman's body to be able to carry out this complex menstrual cycle, her body has to undergo puberty.

REACHING PUBERTY

Puberty describes the changes in body form, hormone levels and behaviour in both boys and girls. Two years before any other hormones start being produced by the body, the hormone dehydroepiandrostenedione (DHEA) is released from the adrenal glands. This process, known as adenarche, usually starts the growth of both pubic and underarm hair.

Once a girl reaches 30 kg of body weight, the body begins to release a hormone from a part of the brain known as the hypothalamus. The hypothalamus is often referred to as the master controller, and plays a key role in co-ordinating many bodily functions such as regulating body temperature, metabolic rate, appetite, water balance, sleep patterns and our response to stress.

The hormone it starts to release at this stage is called Gonadotrophin Releasing Hormone (GnRH). This is released initially at night into small blood vessels that carry GnRH from the hypothalamus to the pituitary gland, a small gland at the base of the brain which is responsible for sending out many different hormone messengers which are essential for growth and other bodily functions.

In the pituitary, GnRH stimulates the release of the two gonadotrophic hormones: follicle stimulating hormone (FSH) and luteinizing hormone (LH).

FSH and LH begin stimulating the ovaries to make oestrogen (see Figure 5). The process of puberty, with the development of breasts, the growth of pubic hair, the height growth spurt and the onset of the first period, takes about four years to complete.

This awakening of the hypothalamo-pituitary-ovarian pathway cannot take place unless the girl has reached a certain weight. For a girl to start her periods she needs to weigh about 47 kg. This is thought to explain why women in the 1830s, who usually got less good food than women today, started their periods at an average age of 17 years, whereas the current average age in the Western world is 13 years. Nutrition plays a vital role in preparing the body for puberty – malnutrition is associated with a delay in the start of a girl's periods, called menarche, while childhood obesity often brings on periods earlier than might be expected.

Once a woman starts her periods, her body needs GnRH to be released from the hypothalamus in order to maintain a regular menstrual cycle. Things that upset this release can affect the menstrual cycle. Two good examples of this are stress and changes in body weight. At a time of acute stress such as studying for exams, a young woman may commonly miss a period.

Women who lose too much weight, such as anorexics, and bring their body weight below 47 kg will often stop menstruating entirely. But women who suddenly change their body weight, whether this is due to a large weight gain or loss, can also experience a change in their usual menstrual cycle.

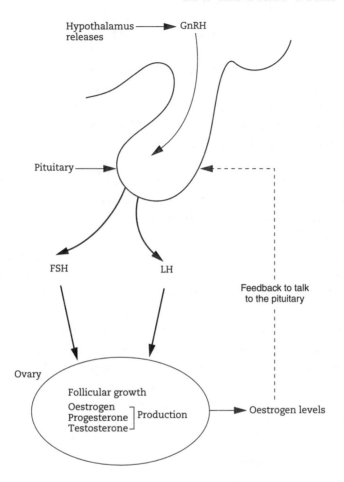

Figure 5

These examples are thought to be the result of a failure in the hypothalamus to release GnRH. This is the body's inbuilt mechanism to ensure that fertilization and pregnancy only happen when the mind and body of the woman can support the pregnancy.

HOW HORMONES WORK IN A NORMAL MONTHLY CYCLE

The menstrual cycle is usually about 28 days long, but may vary in length by a day or two either side. The menstrual cycle involves the interplay between the hypothalamus, the pituitary and the ovaries, and the hormones they produce. Hormones take signals from one part of the body to another, normally through the bloodstream.

The menstrual cycle can be broken down into two halves: the *follicular* (or proliferative) phase, before ovulation, and the *luteal* (or secretory) phase that occurs after ovulation (see page 24).

Throughout the month a number of the dormant eggs in the ovary start to grow. Each egg is surrounded by a number of cells that make a small amount of fluid, producing a very small cyst or follicle (see Figure 6).

We are not sure what triggers the eggs to restart their development after puberty, but if the triggering occurs just after a period, when there are low levels of both FSH and LH being produced by the pituitary, the eggs will be encouraged to continue their growth. Those eggs that recommence their growth at other times of the menstrual cycle will not have the correct hormonal environment and cannot continue to grow.

The Follicular Phase

In the first or follicular phase of the cycle, the hypothalamus sends GnRH to the pituitary. This triggers the pituitary gland to release low levels of follicle-stimulating hormone (FSH). It is this hormone that stimulates the follicles in the ovary to continue to ripen their eggs.

During this time one of the follicles will normally become the dominant follicle, the one most likely to produce a mature egg. The others soon realize they are not going to win the race and stop developing, allowing the dominant follicle to mature.

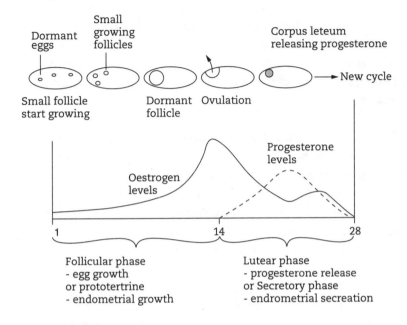

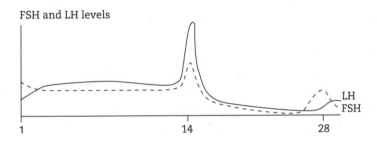

Figure 6

This follicle will grow to a size of 20 millimetres. Then the egg within the follicle is released, in preparation for fertilization. If two, or very rarely more, follicles are evenly grown at this stage of their development it is possible for them all to become dominant. They will all move on to the next stage when ovulation will occur and each follicle's eggs are released. This is one of the causes of multiple pregnancies.

As well as providing a home for the ripening eggs, the follicles in the ovary make and release the hormone oestrogen. During the follicular phase of egg growth the increasing amounts of oestrogen cause the womb lining (endometrium) to start thickening in preparation for a fertilized egg.

To make oestrogen the follicles also require a small amount of the hormone luteinizing hormone (LH). The LH causes the ovary cells directly surrounding the follicle (the thecal cells) to manufacture testosterone. The testosterone is then transported to the cells on the inside of the follicle (the granulosa cells). Here an enzyme converts the testosterone into oestrogen. As the follicle grows in size, stimulated by FSH, the amount of oestrogen produced increases.

Around the middle of the menstrual cycle, when levels of oestrogen are high enough, the pituitary gland produces a large amount or surge of LH. Within 36 hours of the LH surge, the matured follicle in the ovary bursts and releases its egg, a process called ovulation. The egg is collected by one of the Fallopian tubes and transported towards the womb or uterus.

The Luteal Phase

After release of the egg from the follicle at ovulation in the middle of the menstrual cycle, the cells from the burst follicle collapse to form a new cyst called the *corpus luteum* (a Latin term that means 'yellow body'). The corpus luteum now produces progesterone as the main hormone in the second half of the menstrual cycle.

Progesterone causes the thickened lining of the womb to secrete nutrients ready to receive the fertilized egg. These nutrients are designed to feed the growing embryo until the placenta is developed and the mother's blood supply can take over and be used to support the rest of the baby's growth during the pregnancy. This is why it is so important to prepare your body for a pregnancy, because the newly-formed embryo must grow using the nutrients that have been stored within the womb. If this store is poor or deficient, then this will affect the baby's early development. This is the time when pregnancy loss or miscarriage is most common.

At this halfway point in the menstrual cycle there are two options: a sperm will find its way to the egg travelling down the Fallopian tube and fertilize it. In this case the fertilized egg can travel to the womb where it snuggles into the womb lining (the endometrium) in a process called implantation. There the embryo can develop into a foetus. If fertilization occurs, the embryo sends another message back to the corpus luteum in the ovary to let it know it is there. If the corpus luteum receives this message it will continue to produce both progesterone and oestrogen until the placenta has developed. The placenta then takes over the production of these hormones for the rest of the pregnancy.

Alternatively, if fertilization does not take place, after 14 days the corpus luteum begins to shrivel and stops producing progesterone and oestrogen. Levels of the body's oestrogen and progesterone then fall and the thickened womb lining starts to break down and is shed, as a period.

At this point the whole process starts all over again.

WHAT IS DIFFERENT IN A PCOS CYCLE?

The polycystic ovary tends to be larger than the normal ovary because of the cysts. It seems that as the small follicles develop within the ovary of women with PCOS, something interferes with their growth. These partially-developed follicles are the cysts that can be seen by ultrasound in women with PCOS.

The outer coat of the ovary (the tunica) is thickened, as is the tissue within the core of the ovary, the stroma. The thickened core or stroma contains the thecal cells and is responsible for producing extra amounts of testosterone. Testosterone, the 'male' sex hormone, is produced in both men and women, but men produce about 10 times as much as women. As we will see later, excessive production of this hormone in women has a crucial role in the development of many of the symptoms of polycystic ovary syndrome. Although many women with polycystic ovary syndrome produce extra testosterone, the levels are still much lower than those found in men. Despite the fact that women with PCOS may produce a greater amount of testosterone than women with normal ovaries and it is the most common hormonal abnormality detected, by no means do all women with PCOS have a raised testosterone level.

The other hormone that is also commonly elevated and can be suggestive of PCOS is luteinizing hormone (LH). This hormone is produced by the pituitary gland in the brain. We will describe its function in more detail when we look at the control of the normal ovarian function in a later chapter.

The menstrual cycle in women with PCOS is often irregular. The reason for this is thought to be that normal follicular growth and development are interfered with.

There is a great deal of debate about the exact mechanism of the interference. An elevation of the production of testosterone within the ovary has been suggested to be partly responsible. Whatever the mechanism, the interference means that a follicle does not always become dominant and so get to ovulate. Without ovulation the corpus luteum is not formed and the follicles continue to produce a small amount of oestrogen, but no progesterone. The oestrogen continues to drive the growth of the lining of the womb, so that the body effectively stays in the follicular or proliferative phase of the menstrual cycle.

Obviously this pattern could continue for many months, and for some women with PCOS this is exactly what happens. They may go for 2 to 12 months or more without a period. For other women the lining of the womb, which has become slightly overgrown, begins to break down of its own accord. They will experience this as 'spotting', or bleeding between a normal period. Eventually either a follicle does manage to develop and ovulation occurs, so the cycle is re-established, or a period starts although there has been no ovulation, and a new cycle begins.

These irregular cycles and delay or intermittent failure of ovulation is responsible for the problems in conceiving that can be experienced by women with PCOS.

However, not all women with polycystic ovaries have irregular cycles. For some, although it appears that some of the follicles are stopped from developing normally, enough follicles do develop and ovulation occurs without a problem. This explains why many women with polycystic ovaries can conceive naturally.

YOUR QUESTIONS ANSWERED

Is it possible to have a regular menstrual cycle and still not ovulate?

This is certainly possible, and is not confined only to women with PCOS.

All women at the start and end of their reproductive life have what are called 'anovular cycles'. These cycles appear pretty normal in length, but there is a failure of ovulation. This failure is normally identified by measuring the levels of the hormone progesterone in the middle of the second half of the cycle, the luteal phase. It is thought that the follicle develops, but that the process of ovulation and formation of the corpus luteum is poor, resulting in less progesterone production. There is normally sufficient progesterone to allow the cycle to continue so it is not greatly irregular. However, when we look carefully at these cycles we see that they are commonly slightly shorter or longer than normal. These small variations may often go unnoticed by a woman.

What Causes PCOS?

In 1935, when PCOS was first described as a condition, there was great debate as to what caused it. Stein and Leventhal thought it was probably due to 'hormonal stimulation', possibly from the pituitary gland.

The truth is that even now, over 60 years later, no one is quite sure what causes PCOS. Increasingly there are thought to be a number of underlying genetic predispositions (handed down through the family) that determine not just whether a woman develops polycystic ovaries or not, but also what type and how severe her symptoms will be.

As we will see, PCOS is a complex disorder in which a number of factors produce the polycystic ovary and trigger or exacerbate the symptoms which women with PCOS develop.

It is the genes controlling both androgen and insulin production that seem to play the main role in PCO/S. However, there are a number of other genetic factors that will affect the type and severity of symptoms experienced.

Finally, over this web of genetic interactions and predispositions, environmental issues such as diet, pollution, stress levels and how much exercise we take also play important roles in the development (and control of) symptoms.

PCOS is not a simple problem. In this chapter we will take a look at some of the main medical theories that have led us to our current understanding. To do this we will look at various scientific developments that have taken place. Each step along the way has played its part in our present knowledge, and since the story is not finished we will also look at where we are now and where new information is taking us.

In Chapter 2 we looked at the main symptoms of PCOS. Just to recap:

❋   menstrual disturbances including irregular periods, no periods, and irregular spotting (often described as dysfunctional uterine bleeding)

❋   infertility and recurrent miscarriage

❋   symptoms of excess androgens (male hormones), particularly testosterone, excess facial and body hair (hirsutism), acne and hair loss from the scalp, baldness (or alopecia)

❋   obesity

The long-term associated problems or consequences of PCOS include:

❋   increased incidence of endometrial cancer

❋   increased incidence of hypertension

❋   increased incidence of diabetes

❋   increased risk of heart disease

The 'biochemical markers' – signs in the body that PCOS may be present – include:

❋   elevation of testosterone levels

❋   elevation of luteinizing hormone (LH) levels together with normal or low follicle stimulating hormone (FSH) levels

❋   low level of sex-hormone-binding globulin

❋   elevation of insulin levels

❋   abnormal lipid (blood fats) profiles

In the 1960s a new type of blood test, radio-immuno assay, was developed which allowed doctors to test for blood levels of single specific hormones.

For the first time this allowed relatively quick and simple measurements of the hormones LH and FSH, both important in the menstrual cycle.

TOO MUCH LUTEINIZING HORMONE?

Women with classic PCOS, having irregular periods and signs of excess testosterone production (such as hirsutism and acne) were found to have a higher level of LH in their blood, and normal or marginally low levels of FSH. This initially led investigators to suggest that PCOS may be due to a disorder within the controlling hypothalamo-pituitary glands in the brain.

Figure 7 summarizes the hypothalamo-pituitary axis control of the ovary, showing how the ovary produces oestrogen.

As we saw in Chapter 3, Gonadotrophin Releasing Hormone (GnRH) produced by the hypothalamus causes the pituitary to release both LH and FSH. The LH stimulates the thecal cells in the ovary to produce testosterone, which in a normal cycle is converted to oestrogen by the granulosa cells of the follicle.

It was suggested that too much LH might account for the increased production of testosterone in women with PCOS. It was also suggested that higher levels of LH could interfere with the development of the egg within the ovarian follicles. The LH surge is required to allow the immature egg to complete its final cell-division process in preparation for ovulation – but if levels are already high, this cell-division may not take place.

In cases where ovulation did finally take place, it has been suggested that if there were an extended time between the egg 'ripening' and being released, the egg might be prematurely aged and a resulting embryo could be abnormal and be miscarried.[1]

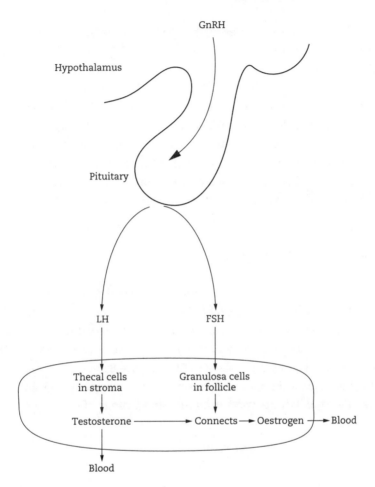

Figure 7

This theory – that PCOS was caused by faulty levels of LH and FSH – does offer us an explanation for the lack of ovulation, higher levels of testosterone and the symptoms of acne and excess body hair that can occur, and the higher rates of miscarriage in women with PCOS.

However, this theory does not explain the common occurrence of obesity, insulin resistance and abnormal blood fat profiles also found in many women with PCOS. There are also women with PCOS who do not have a raised level of LH.

The weight of evidence, at present, suggests that the inappropriate LH secretion is usually a consequence, rather than the cause, of PCOS and its symptoms.

An elevated LH can, however, be a useful marker for predicting women who are at risk of miscarriage. Work by Professor Regan has demonstrated that the rate of miscarriage in women with a normal LH was 7 per cent, compared to 67 per cent in those with an elevated LH.[2] Since then, over 80 per cent of women who present with recurrent miscarriage can be identified as having polycystic ovaries.

TOO MUCH TESTOSTERONE?

Work done by Professor Franks has reviewed a good deal of research and recognized that despite the variety of clinical and biochemical profiles in women with polycystic ovaries, an elevation in the blood levels of male hormones, particularly testosterone, was the most common feature. This points to a specific ovarian cause of PCOS.[3] Figure 8 shows a graph plotting the testosterone levels for women with normal ovaries and groups of women with polycystic ovaries and a range of PCOS symptoms.

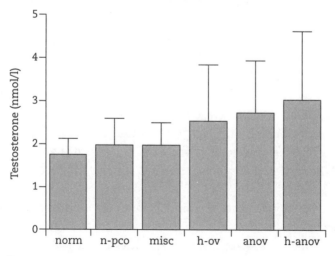

Figure 8

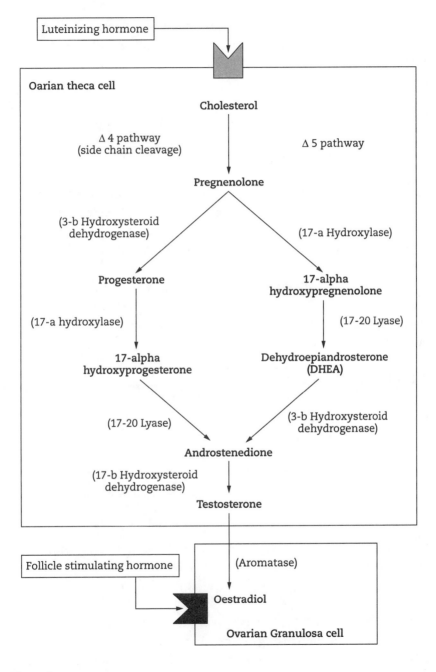

Figure 9

The largest elevation of testosterone is seen in the women with hirsutism and anovulation, but there were elevated levels in all the different groups of women who had polycystic ovaries on ultrasound scan when compared to women with normal ovaries.

This finding led Professor Franks' team to focus on the ovary as the primary cause for the disorder. Figure 9 shows the two-cell biochemical pathway for the manufacture of oestrogen by the ovary.

As we have seen, the ovary's thecal cells produce testosterone, which is usually converted to oestrogen by the granulosa cells of the ovarian follicle. In almost every conversion process such as this one in the body, there is an in-built 'rate-limiting' step which allows the body to regulate the rate of production of the final product by altering the amount of one key enzyme in the pathway. By increasing or decreasing the amount of this key enzyme, it is possible either to speed up or slow down the production of the end product – so, in this case, to increase or reduce the output of testosterone.

A Faulty Link in the Chain?

If the rate of the production of testosterone is increased in women with PCOS, then looking at the rate-limiting step in this pathway would seem a sensible place to start to identify the cause of PCOS. Some work conducted in the US has pointed to an enzyme which catalyses (kick-starts) two enzymic reactions: the 17α-hydroxylase and the 17-20 lyase (see Figure 9).[4,5,6]

If an elevation in testosterone is the cause of PCOS and its symptoms, and the rate-limiting step is known, the question is: What goes wrong with this step?

It is well known that PCOS has a tendency to run in families. In 1991, the Franks team set about looking at a number of large families to see, first, if PCOS is an inherited disease passing from one generation to the next, and secondly, if it is inherited, then is the rate-limiting enzyme or the gene that coded for it different in some way in women who do not suffer from PCOS?

Large families where many of the women family members were affected were identified, and the initial family studies suggested that polycystic ovaries were inherited as 'an autosomal-dominant condition'.[7] This means that the gene responsible is on a chromosome *other* than the sex chromosome – that is, an autosome – and that an affected parent carrying the gene will pass it on to approximately half of their children.

And how were the men in these families affected? The researchers proposed that the male counterpart to polycystic ovaries in women was premature male-pattern baldness. This was defined as significant hair loss before the age of 30.

At last it seemed like the scientists were on to something. But, as with the investigation of most complex diseases, things were not destined to be straightforward.

The gene encoding the 17α-hydroxylase and the 17-20 lyase enzyme, the rate-limiting step, was carefully studied and excluded as the primary cause for PCO and PCOS.[8, 9] It looked like everyone was back to the drawing board.

INSULIN PROBLEMS

In the meantime, other investigators were considering why many women with PCOS also had elevated levels of the hormone insulin.

What Is Insulin and What Does It Do?

Insulin is a peptide hormone (a small protein made from a string of amino acids) that is made by the pancreas. It controls blood sugar levels by allowing the cells to take up and use glucose. The liver (and muscle) cells use glucose and make glycogen. Glycogen is a long branching chain of glucose, and functions as a storage molecule. When your glucose levels start to fall an hour or so after eating, the glycogen is broken down to release glucose back into the bloodstream.

The reason why we need to control our blood glucose levels carefully is that our brains have an absolute requirement for glucose. It is almost the only food the brain can use. This is why the control of blood glucose is so crucial.

What happens if blood glucose is not well controlled can be seen in patients with diabetes. If their blood glucose becomes too high they become confused and disorientated; if it falls below the normal range they will become unconscious.

Every time we eat we challenge this control mechanism. If during a meal you eat more carbohydrate (glucose) than can be stored by the liver and the muscles, the excess is converted and stored as fat. The fat cannot be converted back into glucose but is a very good energy reserve for many cells.

What Are Hyperinsulinaemia and Insulin Resistance?

Hyperinsulinaemia literally means high levels of insulin in the blood.

Insulin resistance describes what happens to the cells that the insulin talks to. When cells become insulin-resistant, they seem to become 'hard of hearing' or resistant to insulin's message. To hear the message, the body has to turn up the volume. It does this by increasing the amount of insulin the pancreas makes for a given amount of glucose in the blood. While the pancreas can still cope with the extra work, normal circulating glucose levels are maintained but at higher levels of insulin. If the pancreas stops being able to produce these higher levels of insulin, initially there is impaired glucose tolerance, when glucose levels are higher than normal after eating. Subsequently, diabetes mellitus ensues.

Could Hyperinsulinaemia Be Responsible for PCOS?

In 1980, the researcher Burghen described the association between high levels of insulin and PCOS.[10] Subsequently, Dr Chang and others found that there was an association between the levels of insulin and the levels of testosterone in women with a normal body weight and PCOS.[11] This was the beginning of the search to see if hyperinsulinaemia caused the elevated testosterone in women with PCOS.

There have been many studies conducted in the area. The conclusion from these is that, in the ovary, insulin appears to stimulate androgen production.[12]

Things all looked very exciting again. Insulin also causes the liver to make less of the steroid hormone-carrier molecule – sex hormone binding globulin (SHBG – see Figure 10).

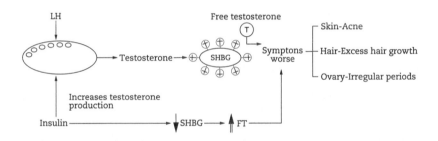

Figure 10

Testosterone made by the ovary is mainly carried in the blood by SHBG. SHBG carries the testosterone much like a car transporter might carry cars on the road. If you imagine a situation where almost all cars were always carried by car transporters, whenever there was room available, there would be few 'free' cars out on the roads. If the number of transporters were to then decrease, the number of free cars driving on the roads would increase greatly. This is much like the situation for testosterone. As the levels of SHBG fall in the blood, the free testosterone – that portion that is available to bind to receptors around the body and cause problems – is greatly increased.

Insulin levels and body weight greatly effect the production of SHBG. As your body weight and insulin levels increase, the levels of SHBG go down.

So insulin has two sites of action: it (along with LH) stimulates an increase in the ovarian manufacture of testosterone, and it decreases the levels of the carrier protein, SHBG, both of which will result in more free testosterone and a potential worsening of symptoms.

However, the insulin theory also had some problems with it. Among other findings, fasting insulin levels were only elevated in one-third of lean women and three-quarters of obese women with PCOS, rather than in all the women with PCOS. The elevated insulin levels found in these women probably does promote testosterone production by the ovary and contributes to the menstrual disturbances that are more common in hyperinsulinaemic women, but is probably not the single cause of the problem.

GENES ASSOCIATED WITH PCOS

From the original family studies completed by the Franks team it was becoming obvious that, although there may be a 'dominant' type of inheritance of PCO, more than one gene would be involved as a cause. The Franks team went on to look at a number of other potential candidate genes.[13]

Looking again at the biosynthetic pathways that produce testosterone, additional work became available suggesting that the enzyme catalysing the first step into the pathway was more likely to be the new rate-limiting step. This reaction converts cholesterol into pregnenolone (see Figure 3) and is catalysed by the P450 side-chain-cleavage enzyme encoded by the gene CYP11a.

Dr Gharani and colleagues went on to demonstrate that, in women with PCO, this gene is associated with elevations of the levels of testosterone.[14] These data indicated that CYP11a is a major susceptibility site for hyperandrogenaemia (excess of male hormones) in women with PCOS, and probably interacts with other genes and the environment to produce the final clinical picture.

As we have seen, hyperinsulinaemia and insulin resistance are very common findings in women with PCOS who present with irregular menstrual cycles and anovulation. Franks' group looked at the gene that codes for insulin. They found that there was a strong association between a specific variation in the insulin gene and anovulation in women with PCOS.[15]

Assuming a dominant mode of inheritance with male pattern baldness as the male counterpart, the data suggested that the insulin gene was involved. Unfortunately the families studied were not quite large enough to confirm this suggestion completely. Franks' team proposed that this variation in the insulin gene results in an oversecretion of insulin from the beta-cells of the pancreas. This, then, may increase testosterone production and, on its own or in combination with other genes, cause PCOS, particularly when anovulation is a feature of the syndrome.

Another consequence of hyperinsulinaemia is the associated risk of developing non-insulin-dependent diabetes mellitus (NIDDM). Women diagnosed as having anovulatory PCOS before menopause are seven times more likely to develop NIDDM later in life, compared to matched controls.[16] This variation in the insulin gene may not only predispose women to anovulatory PCOS, but also to NIDDM.

It has now been suggested that two genes may be required to develop anovulation. The first, possibly CYP11a, causes the characteristic polycystic ovarian structure but no insulin resistance. This is typical of women with polycystic ovaries and regular periods but who may be hirsute. The additional presence of the variation of the insulin gene then makes individuals hyperinsulinaemic and results in anovular, irregular menstrual cycles.

This is an interesting suggestion, because women with PCO and regular cycles tend not to be insulin resistant.

We are now becoming aware that there is a group of genes that predispose us to obesity. The discovery of the Leptin gene, which in mice is a major controller of obesity, is a good example of this. There are likely to be a number of other genes that will affect weight control that have yet to be identified in humans.

As discussed earlier in this chapter, hypersecretion of LH is probably an effect of, rather than the cause of PCOS. But in a disorder that is clearly polygenic (where several genes play a role), there is room for a gene that is involved in the control of GnRH secretion by the hypothalamus and has a specific association with recurrent pregnancy loss.

Finally there are obviously ethnic differences in the way various genes are 'expressed'. A good example of this, and a clue to why different women develop different symptoms, is the distribution density of hair follicles over the body.

Women from Japanese origin typically have very few body hair follicles when compared with women from southern Mediterranean or Middle Eastern backgrounds. Problems related to symptoms such as hirsutism may then vary. So a woman of Japanese descent, who has only to remove one or two troublesome hairs, may find this so insignificant that she does not report it or even consider it to be a problem.

OTHER INTERACTIONS: HYPERINSULINAEMIA – OBESITY

Even without the insulin gene variation, excessive calorie intake will cause weight gain. In women with polycystic ovaries this will exacerbate their symptoms, as other factors drive them to become hyperinsulinaemic. Body weight and body fat are two of the most important factors in determining the severity of symptoms experienced by a woman with polycystic ovaries. Obese women with PCOS are more likely to be hirsute, have irregular periods, and suffer both infertility and miscarriage than lean women with PCOS.

How Does Obesity Make Symptoms Worse?

It seems that, regardless of any genetic predisposition associated with the insulin gene, as women with polycystic ovaries put on weight they are more likely to have symptoms, or their symptoms will get worse. As we have described, as you put on weight you become more hyperinsulinaemic.

As your body weight goes up, your levels of insulin will also tend to increase and this drives your SHBG levels down (Figure 11). The drop in SHBG increases the free testosterone level, and as a result your symptoms get worse.

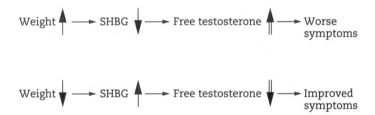

Figure 11

As your body weight reduces these processes can be reversed and your symptoms can improve. There have been many studies to demonstrate that even quite small reductions in body weight result in improvements in both biochemical markers and reproductive function.

Small changes in body weight have a big effect because during the time of weight reduction the individual is much less hyperinsulinaemic.

Avoiding anything that triggers the hyperinsulinaemia is important in helping to manage symptoms.

Are Women with PCOS More Likely to Become Overweight or Obese?

If being overweight is so important in the management of PCOS, surely it should be simple to lose a little weight and improve the symptoms?

This is more straightforward, of course, if the tendency to put on weight is not in some way linked to the underlying problem. Unfortunately, weight gain is thought to be part of the problem. Women with PCOS, whether they are lean or obese, are better able to store the food they eat as a reserve energy supply in the form of body fat. This tendency is greatest in the more overweight women. So not only does being overweight make you more likely to suffer an increasing number and severity of symptoms, but having polycystic ovaries makes you more likely to put on weight. Thus a vicious circle of events is formed that can seem impossible to break.

How Can There Be a Genetic-based Disorder Associated with Infertility?

Normally the basis of evolution is that genetic codes that get passed on are designed to make the species fitter, healthier and more likely to conceive and multiply. So how can PCOS be passed down through the generations? How would women with PCOS ever have managed to pass on their genes to the next generation if they had trouble conceiving? In other words, what possible advantage to the species would there be in having PCOS?

What follows obviously includes a degree of speculation, but it offers us some ideas of where PCOS might have come from and how we may use its potential as an advantage for those who carry the predisposition.

Let's first consider the tendency in women with PCOS to put on weight.

The pressures on modern societies have changed greatly over the last 100 years. Previously many families would have lived through a year when there were times of plenty and other times when food was scarce. The feast-famine communities of the past were common and can still be seen in many areas of the developing world. Under these circumstances, the ability to store more of what we consume as body fat and be more energy-efficient would have offered a considerable advantage. Under these harsh conditions, women with polycystic ovaries would be less likely to drop below the magical 47 kg and so would have remained fertile, while for other women their monthly periods would have ceased, and they would have remained unfertile until they regained weight.

Now consider what has occurred this century, and particularly since the end of the Second World War.

Most of the developed world now lives in a continual state of feast. Luckily, for the majority of us our families do not have times of hardship when food is truly scarce. But for women with polycystic ovaries this might not be such a good thing. They have an evolutionary advantage during times of hardship, but in today's times of excess what was originally an advantage may have become a disadvantage. Getting the balance correct for each individual is very important.

Secondly, let's consider the most common biochemical finding in women with PCOS: an elevated level of serum testosterone. What, if any, evolutionary role could this have played in human development?

Testosterone is the 'male' sex steroid, although it is also made in all women. What role does it serve in women except as a precursor for the production of oestrogen? At present we do not know for sure, however women who undergo hysterectomy and have their ovaries removed at the same time more commonly experience a loss in energy and sex drive post-operatively, despite receiving oestrogen hormone replacement therapy. This can be reversed with the addition of testosterone to the hormone replacement program. It would seem, therefore, that testosterone may affect a woman's energy levels.

There is actually a good animal model for PCOS. It occurs in the spotted hyena. There are female members of the species that look externally similar to the males and distinct from other females. They have been found to have higher levels of male hormones, and their ovaries are said to look remarkably similar to human polycystic ovaries. These 'masculinized' females are more aggressive than the other females of the species and they appear to be better at providing food for their young. This would ensure that their genes stand a better chance of being passed on to the next generation.

So it appears that there may be genetic advantages to having a polycystic ovary predisposition. But it seems likely that today's Western diet and lifestyle may mean that any possible advantages have been temporarily lost.

SECONDARY CAUSES OF PCO/S

No discussion of the causes of PCOS would be complete without a mention of so-called secondary causes. What is meant by secondary causes is that there are a number of recognized conditions in which, on ultrasound, the ovaries look similar to the way they do in women with PCOS.

These secondary causes would include the hormone-secreting abnormalities of the pituitary gland and of the adrenal gland. Similarly, androgen-secreting tumours and severe hyperinsulinaemic conditions need to be excluded before a diagnosis of PCOS can be made with any certainty.

5

How Our Lifestyle Affects PCOS

Stress, pollution and the way we eat all affect PCOS.

As well as the genes for PCOS which we have inherited from our ancestors, there are many things in our day-to-day lives which can make the symptoms of PCOS worse, or push a woman who has PCO (without any symptoms) into developing PCOS (with symptoms).

The positive thing about the fact that what and how we eat, emotional and physical stress, and environmental pollution all play a part in PCOS is that we can control these things. We can't choose our genes, but we can choose what we eat. This chapter explains why these environmental factors do affect PCOS.

MODERN-DAY DIETS

Our diets have changed enormously over the last century, and in particular over the last 40 years. The human race has moved from sparsely populated hunter-gatherer communities to densely populated communities were food is mass produced, refined and processed, mainly to allow a longer shelf-life.

These processing techniques often alter the taste of our food. So manufacturers add chemicals to enhance the 'flavour', or cover the poor taste. Many scientists are now arguing that this highly refined and processed food is low in nutritional value and contains many additives which could be harmful to health. This affects everyone, but is particularly relevant to women with PCOS.

How Is Modern Food Less Nutritious?

Nutrients are not the same as calories. The calorific value of the food we eat refers to the amount of energy we get from it. The nutrient value of the food relates not only to how much protein, carbohydrates and fats it contains, but also its amount of vitamins and minerals. While the calorific value of food may have stayed the same (or even increased for some foods where additional sugar has been added to 'improve' or 'enhance' the taste), the nutrient value has decreased. This loss of nutrients starts with modern farming techniques.

Modern Farming Techniques

Modern techniques are designed to increase the crop yield per unit area of land, making farming more efficient and profitable. Vast amounts of chemical fertilizers which contain the elements nitrogen, phosphorus and potassium have been used to stimulate plant growth. While plants need little more than these elements (along with water, sunlight and carbon dioxide from the atmosphere) for the process known as photosynthesis which they use to live and grow, the same is not true of animals. The use of chemical fertilizers rather than manure, compost and crop-rotation has led to a reduction in the soil mineral content of magnesium, manganese, zinc and copper.[1]

A good example of the effect of soil mineral-deficiency has been seen on the prairie lands of Florida, where the soil now contains so little copper that unless cattle feed is supplemented with copper the cows which feed on the land develop osteoporosis and fractures.[2]

Other elements essential for normal human function which are now at low levels in the soil include boron, chromium, iodine, iron, magnesium and zinc. So modern plant crops and the animals which feed on them cannot contain the best levels of these nutrients because they don't exist in the soil in the first place.

Simple Food Processing

After harvest, many crops are processed ready for storage and to use in making other foodstuffs. For example, a lot of wheat is ground into flour, and refined into white flour, which means the husk is taken out. This is because insects such as weevils feed on the husks but will not be attracted to the flour once they are removed. The bits of the wheat grain which are extracted contain between 70 and 90 per cent of the vitamin and mineral content of the wheat, which is then lost.[3]

What is left has only a poor nutritional value and is good at making people fat, as we will see later. Refined flour, together with refined sugar which has almost no vitamin or mineral content, make up about half the calories in most Western diets, so it is easy to see how nutritional deficiencies can develop.

Complex Food Processing

Foods that are easily prepared, look enticing and have a prolonged shelf-life are now being made by the food technology industry. Development of these products may involve one or a combination of processing techniques such as bleaching, irradiation, extraction with organic solvents, exposure to extremes of temperature or pH and the addition of other chemicals to preserve, texturize, colour or otherwise modify the food. All these processes have been shown to detract from the nutritional content of the food, while potentially adding to the 'toxic load' that the body has to process.

How Does this Affect Women with PCOS?

Eating less nutritious food cannot be of much benefit to someone who is well and healthy, let alone someone who may have a medical problem or a potential problem.

Scientific evidence about how poor diet affects women with PCOS is scarce – but this is hardly surprising given the small amount of research which has been done on any aspect of PCOS at all.

Which Vitamins and Minerals Are Important for PCOS?

Vitamins and minerals play many roles in the body, and an exhaustive description is beyond the remit of this book.

Vitamins and minerals are commonly used as co-factors for enzyme actions. The formation of insulin is an example, requiring vitamin B_6 and zinc, while chromium improves insulin's efficiency. Chromium levels have been reported to be lower in patients with diabetes.[4] Chromium deficiency is also reported to increase with age.[5] But for most vitamins and minerals, our ability to assimilate them seems to decline as we get older.

Supplementation with chromium has been reported to improve glucose tolerance and lipid profiles (fat levels) in people who do not suffer from diabetes, and reduce insulin requirements in people with diabetes.[6,7,8]

Although these studies were conducted on relatively small numbers of patients, it is likely that chromium is one element that will be seen to be increasingly used to support carbohydrate metabolism in those who require it. Since hyperinsulinaemia and insulin resistance are major factors for developing PCOS, and can be regarded as the very early changes on the road to becoming diabetic, then chromium deficiency may be more important than previously recognized. And chromium is only one of the components of our diet that our bodies require to work properly.

Current figures from the US suggest that as many as 30 per cent of teenage girls and 80 per cent of the institutionalized elderly are nutrition-ally deficient in at least one vitamin or mineral.[9] We cannot assume that today's well-balanced diet will necessarily fulfil all our requirements.

For many women with PCOS, fertility is one of the most important issues. We are now very aware of the benefits of folic acid supplementation in reducing neural tube defects, and more recently we have seen the reduction in risk of pre-eclampsia from supplementation with vitamins E and C during pregnancy.[10] Ensuring that you obtain a diet of high nutritional value will be important not only for your current health, but also for the health of your future children.

POLLUTION IN OUR FOOD AND ENVIRONMENT

There are many groups of chemicals that inadvertently or directly get added to our food, either during the time they are growing or as a consequence of food processing. It has been estimated that since the early 1950s more than 3,500 new man-made chemicals have found their way into the foods we regularly eat.

During growth, plants and animals are exposed to:

✳ Insecticides: organophosphates (linked to Gulf War Syndrome) and nitrates
✳ Pesticides: including DDT, Dinoseb, Ethyl dibromide, Heptachlor, Lindane, pronamide and Methoxychlor, all of which have been cited as probable human carcinogens (cancer-causing agents) by the US Environmental Protection Agency.
✳ Pharmaceutical drugs: anabolic steroids are commonly used as animal growth-promoters in beef and pork production. Antibiotics are used to reduce infection caused by overcrowded rearing conditions. In the US 60 per cent of cattle, over 90 per cent of pork and 95 per cent of poultry have antibiotics routinely added to their feeds.

As a consequence of environmental pollution or food processing, we are also exposed to:

✳ Industrial pollution: Dioxins and PCBs
✳ Plastic components: Alkyphenols, bisphenolics and phthalates

❀ Food additives: The 'E' numbers and sodium (salt). In food processing, additional sodium is added to the food to prolong its shelf-life and improve its taste.

How Do These Chemicals Affect Women with PCOS?

All the chemicals listed above can be considered as anti-nutrients. Our bodies do not want them and have to work hard to process (metabolize) them and get rid of them (detoxify). In order to process them the body uses up vital nutrients.

Many of these chemicals also inhibit or reduce our body's ability to extract and use the vitamins and minerals from our diets, and have been shown to have many other negative health consequences including carcinogenic actions.

To show in more detail how food processing and pollution actually affect women with PCOS directly, we will look at chemicals known as endocrine disrupting chemicals (EDCs), and at salt or sodium (Na). For more in-depth information, turn to the Further Reading chapter.

Endocrine Disrupting Chemicals

Many of the compounds listed in the groups above, including pesticides, fertilizers, industrial pollutants and plastic components, have actions that mimic hormones in the body and are now called 'endocrine disrupting chemicals' (EDCs).

It is likely that if these chemicals affect the oestrogen receptor, some of them will also affect other steroid receptors. This is why, for example, the synthetic progestins that were designed to mimic progesterone in the combined oral contraceptive pill all have slightly different side-effects. The small alterations in the chemical structure of the different progestins turn on or off different progesterone (and other steroid) receptors. These variations in steroid-receptor action are thought to account for the different side-effects that each different chemical progestin produces.

What Are the Effects of EDCs?

In the animal kingdom we have seen some dramatic examples of fish, seals and even polar bears that have been shown to have developed as hermaphrodites (with both male and female sexual organs, simultaneously). This has been directly linked to an increasing exposure to EDCs. These hermaphrodites are thought to be genetically male members of the species, but exposure to 'oestrogen-like' chemicals has caused them to develop some of the female reproductive organs as well as their male organs. Since these chemicals are having profound effects on the biochemistry and sexual make-up within the animal kingdom, it would be foolish to assume that humans will be immune to their effects.

We have seen the documented fall in the male sperm count over the last 50 years, which has been so staggering that doctors have had to reclassify the 'normal' range. Fifteen years ago a normal sperm count was considered to be greater than 60 million sperm per millilitre. Now the normal count is defined as above 20 million sperm per millilitre. Although no cause has been clearly identified in men to account for the decline, it is not unlikely that increased environmental exposure to oestrogenic toxins has some role to play.

In women we have seen an increase in the incidence of hormone-related disorders including menstrual disturbances, fibroids, endometriosis, infertility and breast cancer. The incidence of breast cancer has almost tripled in the last 50 years, from 1 in 22 to 1 in 8 women.

PCOS is an endocrine disorder in which, as we have discussed, there is typically an elevated amount of testosterone that is associated with symptoms such as acne and excess body hair.

The levels of oestrogen in women with PCOS are not usually elevated beyond the normal range. They are usually similar to those seen in the mid-follicular phase of egg development.

As many women with PCOS have an irregular cycle – or, even for those whose cycle is regular, may be anovular (not releasing an egg at ovulation each month) – they are exposed to chronic levels of unopposed oestrogen without the balancing effect of progesterone. The effects of this chronic exposure to oestrogen are:

✳ at the pituitary gland, a feed-back mechanism produces the suppressed levels of FSH commonly seen in women with PCOS
✳ at the endometrium (womb lining), the continuous oestrogen drive, without regular progesterone opposition, increases the long-term risks of developing endometrial cancer, especially in mid- to later life and after menopause. It can sometimes be linked to bleeding after menopause, which is always checked out seriously by doctors. Women with PCOS before menopause can also suffer irregular small bleeds or spotting. This is thought to occur because the endometrium has been stimulated to grow for a prolonged period, becomes overgrown and may then partially break down, resulting in the spotting.
✳ We do not yet know if women with PCOS are of greater risk of developing breast cancer, but as this is also commonly an oestrogen-driven condition this could be a possibility.
✳ Finally, we know that oestrogens are responsible for the fat distribution that is typical of the female shape. We don't know if environmental exposure to chemicals that potentiate the action of the oestrogen produced within a woman's body also causes weight gain, but this may well play a role for some women.

Additional oestrogenic load from our environment may result in a larger number of anovular menstrual cycles and more infertility, more irregular bleeding patterns, an increased risk of endometrial and possibly breast cancer and a greater tendency to lay down body fat.

While it is not currently possible to site double-bind placebo-controlled experiments to confirm that these chemicals are adding to the endocrine load for women with PCOS, on balance we would suggest that taking measures to avoid EDCs seems sensible.

Salt

Salt (or sodium) is essential for life, so much so that during the time of the pharaohs in Egypt, workers were paid in salt. Since salt has been manufactured we have used it increasingly in food preparation. During food processing additional salt is now commonly added to our food, particularly meat and dairy produce, to preserve and prolong the shelf-life and to 'improve' the flavour of over-processed foods. In the US it is estimated that Americans eat 20 times more salt than they require.[11]

The effect of this type of food processing has been to increase dramatically the amount of sodium we consume, reversing the sodium (Na):potassium (K) ratio from 1Na:7K to 3.6Na:K. The result of this excess sodium in our diets is an increase in the incidence of high blood pressure (hypertension), and is thought to account for about one-third of the hypertensive disease that requires treatment. High blood pressure is one of the main risk factors for developing heart disease and is also more common in women with PCOS. Eating processed foods with a hidden salt content can therefore add to the risks of high blood pressure and heart disease for women with PCOS.

HOW WHAT WE EAT AFFECTS OUR BODIES

The food that we eat contains three major groups of molecules: protein, fats, and carbohydrates.

Proteins are made from strings of amino acids, the building-blocks that are coded for by our DNA. These proteins are used by our bodies to build most cell structures. Muscle cells have a particularly high protein content.

Fats have a number of roles within our bodies' cells, for example they form part of the double layer of cell membranes. A number of specific fats are used as the basis of hormone structures such as the sex steroids and the prostaglandins. Therefore, the types of fats we eat may affect our cell membranes and our hormones. Changes in dietary fat types and amounts have important implications in the management of women with PCOS, as we will discuss later. The other main role of body fat is as an energy-storage molecule.

Carbohydrates are the body's main immediate source of energy, and although the body can run on protein and fat, as in times of hardship or fasting, it is less efficient at this. The body's first choice will always be to use carbohydrates.

Carbohydrate Metabolism

Most of the carbohydrates found in nature are complex, or treated like complex carbohydrates by our bodies. Complex carbohydrates (starches) are long strings of sugar molecules (glucose) that are stored within the cells of plants. Complex carbohydrates are found in green and root vegetables, beans, lentils and whole grains. The cell wall of these foods must be broken down to allow the starch to be digested to release the sugar and its potential energy. These processes take time and release sugar into the bloodstream slowly. These foods also contain non-digestible carbohydrate or fibre, mainly from the cell walls, which does not get absorbed and passes though the digestive tract, keeping it running smoothly. Although we cannot digest the fibre ourselves, the friendly bacteria that live within our large bowel (the colon) rely on this for food. We, in turn, rely on these good bacteria to stop other less friendly bacteria from multiplying.

The simple carbohydrates found in nature are mainly contained within fruits as fructose. Fructose is a small molecule and needs no digestion, so once released from the fruit can be absorbed rapidly. The body cannot use it directly and it must be converted to glucose by the liver. This effectively slows down the effect this sugar has on our metabolism. There is some glucose found in fruits such as bananas and grapes. This will result in a more rapid rise in blood glucose levels.

As we can see from this, most of the carbohydrates we have been eating for centuries contain sugars that are released into our blood system relatively slowly, and are in foods that contain many vitamins and minerals our bodies need.

Carbohydrates in Processed Foods

Refined carbohydrates contain the sugar molecule glucose. The process of refinement has aided the digestive process by breaking down the cell walls of the plants and releasing the starch, and sometimes also breaking down the complex starch molecule into smaller carbohydrates or glucose. When eaten, refined carbohydrates have the same effect on the blood's glucose levels as refined sugar does. They cause a very rapid rise in the blood sugar.

The brain uses blood glucose for its source of energy. Your brain needs blood sugar levels to be very well controlled within a narrow normal range. If blood glucose is taken outside this normal range, and our body cannot deal with it, as in people with diabetes, illness and even death can occur. When the blood glucose level is too high the person with diabetes will become confused and disorientated; if the level falls too low the person will rapidly become unconscious.

This is why the body has developed an elaborate set of mechanisms to maintain the status quo every time we eat a meal.

How Your Body Controls Blood Sugar

Insulin is the hormone that regulates blood sugar levels. When we eat we need to release the correct amount of insulin so that our blood glucose levels remain within the normal range. If we release too much insulin we will rapidly push the blood glucose levels too low (becoming hypoglycaemic). If we release too little insulin we will become hyperglycaemic, with too much blood sugar circulating.

The body regulates the amount of insulin released dependent on the rate of absorption of glucose. Consider what happens when we eat a meal of mainly complex carbohydrate – a bean and lentil salad for example. It is digested first to allow the glucose to be absorbed.

The rate of glucose absorption will depend on how much we have eaten at the meal. If we have eaten a small meal there will be a slow absorption of glucose, and only a small amount of insulin will be needed to control the challenge. If we eat a very large meal then there will be a more rapid absorption of glucose which will require a larger amount of insulin.

When we eat refined carbohydrates and sugar there is a very rapid rise of blood glucose, even for only a small number of calories. These need only to be absorbed, rather than having to be digested first and then absorbed like complex carbohydrates. The rapid rate of absorption causes the body to make a large amount of insulin. This results in a larger insulin production than would be seen for the same number of calories from a complex carbohydrate source.

Our modern diets – which consist mainly of refined carbohydrates and a high level of processed sugars – are effectively driving all of us to become mildly hyperinsulinaemic. As a result, an increasing number of people are becoming overweight and developing diabetes.

Insulin drives glucose into the cells, to avoid blood sugar levels becoming too high and negatively affecting our brain's function. Initially the insulin will drive glucose into the liver and muscles, where it is stored as glycogen. Once these stores have been topped up, the rest is converted into a type of fat known as a triglyceride, which can then be taken up by fat cells and stored as body fat. A refined carbohydrate diet used to be recommended for people with diabetes, until it was realized that while this *seemed* to control their blood glucose levels, it resulted in very abnormal blood fat levels that greatly predisposed them to cardiovascular disease.

Immediately after eating sweets and sugar that contain no fat we can demonstrate a rise in the blood fat levels, especially triglycerides. These fats not only get deposited within the blood vessels, increasing our risk of cardiovascular disease, but will also be laid down as additional body fat.

When we consider the problems encountered by women with PCOS, we know that they need to avoid anything that will cause them to become either more hyperinsulinaemic or overweight. A typical modern diet, where more than 50 per cent of the calories now comes from refined carbohydrates and sugar, will certainly make a woman with PCOS suffer worse symptoms, or push a woman with PCO into developing PCOS.

Low Carbing

I would like to lose weight to help improve my symptoms. I have read about Barry Sears and Dr Atkins' diets, which involve avoiding carbohydrates. Should I try a low-carbohydrate diet?

There has been a lot written over the last few years about 'low carbing'.

The concept of reducing your carbohydrate intake comes from the knowledge that if you consume some protein with everything you eat, you will reduce the amount of insulin your body produces. Low stable blood insulin levels will reduce the drive to convert carbohydrates into fat.

However, there are a few important points to remember.

The positive effect of eating protein at each meal is greatly reduced if you eat it with refined carbohydrates. As we have suggested, you should stop eating refined carbohydrates and replace them with complex carbohydrates, particularly those obtained from vegetables or a variety of wholegrains, not just wheat. When you start to eat some protein with every meal, you will find that you eat fewer carbohydrates because protein is better at making you feel full.

What Barry Sears actually recommends is eating 1 ounce of protein for every 2 ounces of carbohydrate. This is not avoiding carbohydrates; on the contrary he suggests you eat twice as much carbohydrate as protein. The best ratio to stabilize insulin levels is 1:1.7, though this obviously takes some working out in everyday life.

What happens when you cut out almost all carbohydrates from your diet?

Carbohydrates are a good source of energy and almost an absolute requirement for your brain. And your body is immensely resourceful. If you feed it only protein for a while, it will adapt to the challenge. Your body can convert the protein into carbohydrate to keep your blood glucose levels stable and feed your brain. This is more energy-intensive for the body and may result in fewer excess calories being stored as fat. But the conversion of protein to carbohydrates will also produce much more of the toxic waste ammonia, which your kidneys will have to remove. This will put an extra strain on your kidneys and, if you had any pre-existing kidney damage, could be dangerous. Certainly those with poor kidney function are often put on low protein diets, to protect their kidneys from this type of damage.

Since many women's diets are actually heavily laden with carbohydrates and very little protein, the change to eating some protein with every meal and cutting back on carbohydrate intake – especially when combined with changing from refined to complex carbohydrates – may be helpful, but this is not low carbing, it is just achieving more of a balance.

Moving to a very low carb diet is not a good idea, because you will start to lose the goodness that comes from the many vitamins, minerals and fibre content of vegetables.

Also, we do not believe in the concept of dieting, as the very term implies something not sustainable in the longer term, and so your weight and symptoms will fluctuate. Moving to a balanced, healthy way of eating will allow you to maintain your success for the long term, safely.

How Dietary Fats Affect Your Body

Body fat is your body's main fuel reserve. However, you do not need to eat fat to store extra calories. As we saw earlier, any extra sugar that is consumed will be converted to fat for storage. There is actually a vast excess of calories stored as body fat. For a slim woman who weighs 10 stone 10 (150 lb/68 kg) and is 20 per cent body fat, she will store 10 per cent of her fat (1.1 stones/15 lb/6.8) as an energy reserve. This represents 61,200 calories of stored energy, and is sufficient energy to complete four marathons without recharging the energy supply! We all stock a vast excess of energy as fat. So even a very thin person will not run out of body fat as an energy store.

There are three main types of fat:

1   essential fats
2   non-essential fats
3   trans fats.

Essential Fats

There are two essential fats. Also known as essential fatty acids (EFAs), they are two long-chain fatty acids that your body cannot make: linoleic acid (omega-6 series) and alpha-linolenic acid (omega-3 series). These unsaturated fatty acids must be obtained from your diet.

Good sources of both the omega-3 and omega-6 fatty acids include flaxseed (linseed) oil, pumpkin seeds and soya. The omega-6 fatty acids are used to make arachidonic acid, whereas the omega-3 series go on to make EPA and then DHA.

The omega-3 fatty acids (especially EPA and DHA) are vital for normal brain development and functioning. Rich sources of EPA and DHA can be found in oily fish such as mackerel, sardines and, to a lesser degree, salmon. So there is some truth in the old wives' tale that eating fish can make you brainy!

The omega-3 fatty acids are also the building-blocks for another group of chemical messengers call prostaglandins. The omega-3 series of prostaglandins have been found to reduce the risk of heart disease, stroke and non-insulin-dependent diabetes, all of which are more common in women with PCOS. They also tend to be anti-inflammatory, reducing the risk of arthritis.

The omega-6 prostaglandins seem to counteract the good effects of the omega-3 prostaglandins.

Our modern diets have tended to favour the omega-6 series rather than the omega-3 series. The ratio of 3 series:6 series has moved from 2:1 a few hundred years ago to 1:7 in most modern diets. It has been suggested that this change is responsible in part for the increasing incidence of heart disease and the other conditions mentioned above. So it is important to look at the types of fats you are eating.

Non-essential (Saturated) Fats

Saturated fats are again long chains of carbon atoms, where hydrogen atoms have saturated all the available spaces and there are no double bonds present.

Saturated fats are found in animal products and are the main fat in palm and coconut oils. Not having double bonds present makes these fats tend to be solid rather than liquid. This is reflected in their effect on the cell membrane – they decrease their fluidity of the membrane. This affects how the cell and its receptors may function.

Saturated fats increase your risk of developing heart disease and their intake should be moderated.

Trans Fats

If natural fats are processed by heat or hydrogenation (to turn liquid fats into solids, as in some margarines, for example), their atomic structure is altered to form what are known as trans fats. All processed oils contain trans fats; the more solid the oil, the higher the amount. Liquid vegetable oils typically contain 6 per cent, while margarines can contain up to 58 per cent. On the label you can identify the trans fats as they are also called hydrogenated or partially hydrogenated fats. Hydrogenated fats should by law be clearly indicated on the label.

The altered trans fats in the diet make their way into cell membranes in the same way as natural fats, but they alter the function of the membranes. In many ways trans fats can be considered like saturated fatty acids, in that our bodies do not know how to use them, and they should be avoided.

Trans fats cause an increase in cholesterol levels in the body. This is particularly true of the low-density lipoproteins (LDLs). Too many LDLs will increase your risk of heart disease.

EXERCISE

Our increasingly sedentary lifestyle plays a major part in our increasing obesity. We are seeing the effects of a lack of physical exercise in younger and younger people. One in three Americans is now overweight, and at least one in four is considered obese. This trend is growing throughout Europe and the rest of the Western world.

A recent report in the *British Medical Journal* found that the incidence of both overweight and obese children aged 4 years has increased from 5 per cent (overweight) and 15 per cent (obese) in 1990 to 7.6 per cent and 20.3 per cent respectively in 1999.[12] The criterion for obesity used in this report was very conservative, and so this is probably an underestimate of the real magnitude of the problem. There were no differences in the incidence between boys and girls; these data are consistent with the evidence of an epidemic of adult obesity and support the view that prevention needs to begin in childhood.

Children do less exercise than their parents did when they were young. They get ferried to schools by car rather than going on foot or by bicycle. They also watch more television and take less exercise at home than their parents used to.

A lack of physical exercise has many effects on health. Eating a Western diet and doing no exercise causes muscles and even bones to waste away. This is because physical exercise allows us to maintain or increase our muscle mass. As the intensity of the exercises we perform increases, so does our ability to gain additional muscle mass.

The Benefits of Exercise for Women with PCOS

The benefits of increasing muscle mass or decreasing our percentage of body fat are enormous. Our basal metabolic rate – the rate at which our cells burn fat while at rest – is directly related to our lean body mass. As our lean body mass increases, so does our basal metabolic rate. Muscles have been estimated to burn 7 calories per pound of body muscle while at rest. So your muscles are burning up calories while you are at rest or asleep. Fat cells burn no calories. Therefore, the more muscular you are the easier it becomes to stay lean.

The leaner you become, the less body fat you carry and the higher your SHBG (sex hormone binding globulin – see Chapter 4). For women with PCO/S this will reduce the effect of additional testosterone production and minimize symptoms such as acne and hirsutism.

Weight-bearing exercise and cardiovascular fitness have both been demonstrated to improve insulin sensitivity. This means that the fat and muscle cells are more receptive to insulin in the blood, therefore your body pumps out less insulin to get the same response, which means positive changes in both blood sugar and fat lipids. So exercise can be used in the management of hyperinsulinaemia, obesity and PCOS.

Finally, it is worth noting that anabolic steroids, used by both male and female athletes in some cases to improve their performance, work by mimicking the action of testosterone! Women with PCOS may actually, because of their naturally elevated levels of testosterone, not only be more competitive but also may be able to put on additional lean body mass with greater ease than women without this predisposition. It could be argued that women with polycystic ovaries are born natural athletes, or even that their bodies demand this of them. Failure to listen to your body's needs could be seen to result in symptoms.

STRESS

There seems little doubt that there is more stress in today's modern society than was present in the past. There are three types of stress: physical stress – such as that experienced during exercise and everyday work – emotional stress, and dietary stress.

Dietary stress is a result of eating refined foods. As we have seen, this causes blood glucose to rise quickly after eating refined carbohydrates, which is followed by a rapid increase in the blood insulin. The insulin causes the glucose to be stored as glycogen or fat. This brings down the blood glucose rapidly.

To counter this rapid fall in blood glucose we release a small amount of the two stress hormones from the adrenal gland: cortisol and adrenaline. These hormones act to increase the blood glucose again. This increases the total stress experienced by your body. Eating complex carbohydrates results in a slower absorption of the glucose and a smaller rise in blood insulin. This means that the swings in blood glucose are not as large and do not result in the same release of the stress hormones.

Whatever the stressor – dietary, emotional or physical – the body responds in the same way, by increasing the production of stress hormones. This mobilizes your glucose stores in preparation to allow you to respond to the stress. These hormones are known as the 'flight or fight' hormones because this is what your body is being prepared to do. The type of stress we would have been under in the not too distant past would have needed us to respond in one of these two ways. Today our stresses are very different, but our bodies respond with the same hormonal release.

So what happens when these stress hormones are released? The extra cortisol is linked to a condition called Cushing's syndrome, when you develop central weight gain (that is, weight is gained around the stomach), depression, insomnia, irregular periods, poor libido, excess body hair and acne, high blood pressure, weakness and diabetes. Sufferers also are insulin resistant. The main cause of the syndrome is the use of steroids to treat other medical conditions, but you can see that many of the same symptoms are those experienced by women who have PCOS.

Stress will cause the extra release of cortisol and adrenaline. When they are not 'used' appropriately the cortisol will tend to drive your body towards the symptoms listed above.

The hyperinsulinaemia and insulin resistance associated with PCOS also have an effect on the adrenal gland's steroid hormone production. The elevated insulin levels commonly seen in women with PCOS have been shown to increase cortisol levels. So women with PCOS who have elevated insulin levels consequently make more cortisol and have an exaggerated cortisol-production response to stress. This is another example of why exercise may be so beneficial. In the absence of good stress management, a hyperinsulinaemic women with PCOS will be further at risk of developing Cushing's syndrome.

Any stress-management regime ideally needs to act on all three types of stress – physical, emotional and dietary. It is not often easy to change the things in your life that are producing physical or emotional stress, but you can go some way towards reducing your total stress by reducing your dietary stress.

Many complementary therapies have been found to reduce the symptoms experienced by women with PCOS. They seem to modulate the body's stress response. This may be part of the action of such diverse therapies such as aromatherapy and massage, meditation and acupuncture, though all may also have other specific actions.

For practical tips on reducing dietary stress see chapters 10 and 11.

EATING DISORDERS

The human race has a complicated interaction with food. Eating means more than just receiving nourishment and nutrients. Much of our social behaviour revolves around eating, and food is commonly used to punish or to comfort. Particularly for those who have a weight-management problem, their interaction with food can be more complicated than just a matter of what and when they eat. They may have patterns of behaviour that are associated with how they were brought up and the way in which food was used during this time. If your mother always sneaked you some chocolate after you had been in trouble, this association can be difficult to change as you get older. In recent studies it is now suggested that women with PCOS have a higher incidence of bulimia nervosa. This is a binge-eating type of behaviour where after overeating a person feels so guilty and full of self-hatred that they make themselves vomit. There is not a reported higher incidence of anorexia in women with PCOS.

Changing the way we eat and approach food will obviously be more difficult for some than for others. Binge eating will tend to drive your body to lay down body fat, and this will make the symptoms of PCOS worse. If you are concerned that binge eating or bulimia is a part of your problem, then getting appropriate help will be very important. When going to see your doctor to talk about getting a diagnosis, or if you know you have polycystic ovaries but have never been able to tell anyone about having an eating problem, you will need to talk to someone. Getting help with the way you use food in your life is as important as eating the right things.

Although less common among women with PCOS, anorexia or intermittent fasting and yo-yo types of diets have a very detrimental effect on health and weight management. If you decide to try and lose weight by fasting during the day and then eating a small meal in the evening – a common technique employed to fit into our social convention of eating our main meal at night – you will fail. The reason is that when you have been asleep all night, on waking your body will be looking to take in some calories. If you decide not to eat your body then has no idea when your next meal is going to be coming along. So your body will attempt to conserve energy. To do this it will tend to suppress your basal metabolic rate (BMR). This is the rate at which your cells burn fuel. In 'fasting time' this is slowed down so that the fuel supplies you have in your body stored as fat can last longer. The problem with decreasing your BMR is that when you do eat next you will then store a greater proportion of what you eat as fat.

Finally, when you fast your body has still to maintain a normal blood glucose to feed your brain. We have developed a number of adapted mechanisms to ensure that we are able to maintain a normal blood glucose level even if we are unable to eat for many days. The main mechanism is to break down our body's muscles and convert the released amino acids from the muscle protein into glucose. You cannot convert fat into glucose. So when you fast you lose your muscles first. Since your muscle or your lean body mass is a major determinant of your BMR, the more muscle you have the greater your BMR, and the less muscle you have the slower your BMR. Fasting and losing muscle further drives down your BMR, and once you start to eat at the end of the day more of your calories will be stored as fat.

The tendency to have little or no breakfast, a small lunch and your main meal in the evening, besides the metabolic effects described, also gives you most of your calories at a time when there is no need for them since you are asleep. As there is no need for them you will store them as more fat. If you are going to eat one meal that is bigger than the other, then breakfast like a king, lunch like a prince and dine like a pauper. But ideally, five evenly-spaced small meals work best.

Long-term Health Consequences

Knowing that you are at a potentially higher risk of developing the following long-term consequences of PCOS may make for dispiriting reading, but please bear in mind that with this knowledge you can choose whether or not you want to take action. Also, life throws up problems for us all – choice is often denied to many people who develop a health condition having had no idea that it could have been on the horizon. Try to see this knowledge as a positive thing.

Having the ability to recognize a part of your genetic predisposition should be seen as a very big advantage. Knowing that you will respond well to an active lifestyle and that the way you choose to eat and live your life will have obvious effects on how you look, feel and function gives you some personal insight, and then a better than average chance of fulfilling your own potential.

Almost all of the associated risks outlined below are long term. This means that there is normally a long period of time between the identification of having PCO/S and the emergence of problems, if they arise at all. This long lead-time gives you the scope to choose and experiment, to a degree, with either continuing down the same path or moving in a slightly new direction. Choosing lifestyle changes that improve symptoms in the short term will help to reduce all the long-term risks.

LONG-TERM HEALTH CONCERNS FOR WOMEN WITH PCO/S

Obesity

Women with PCOS are more likely than those without to have weight-management problems. By no means are all women with PCOS overweight. Those who do have a problem with their weight-management are likely to be in the group of women who are also hyperinsulinaemic and insulin resistant. Women with PCOS are more likely to put on weight centrally. An apple shape as opposed to a pear shape.[2]

As we have seen, many women with PCOS who put on weight find their symptoms tend to get worse. Becoming overweight has many other long-term associated problems. It reduces mobility, prolongs healing time, and increases the risks of all the other long-term risk factors identified below. It is therefore important to try and control your weight – with the support of a qualified practitioner, family and friends.

Eating Disorders

As many as 60 per cent of women with bulimia have been found to have polycystic ovaries. This is much higher than the reported 22 per cent incidence of PCO in the general population. Since many women with PCOS have a problem controlling their weight, this association may not seem surprising. However, attempting to change the way you eat could represent a major difficulty. It would be important for those who have a problem of this nature to seek additional help. Please see the Useful Addresses chapter of this book.

Abnormal Blood Lipid profile

A low level of the 'good' cholesterol – high density lipoprotein (HDL) cholesterol – and an increased level of the 'bad' cholesterol – low density lipoprotein (LDL) – together with high triglyceride levels are seen in the women with PCOS, particularly those who are hyperinsulinaemic and have insulin resistance.[2,3] This situation is associated with both the risk of developing heart disease and non-insulin-dependent diabetes. Healthy eating and exercise can help.

High Blood Pressure

Women with PCOS are four times more likely to suffer from high blood pressure than age- and weight-matched controls.[4] High blood pressure is an independent risk factor for heart disease. Good nutrition, less processed foods containing salt, and exercise can all help with this.

Subfertility

For those women who do not have a regular menstrual cycle, a delay in conceiving is not uncommon. Normally a woman releases an egg every month, offering 12 times in the year when she can conceive. If the number of times ovulation occurs is reduced, then there is less chance to conceive. A few women with PCOS rarely ovulate at all.

A small amount of weight loss has been demonstrated to restart normal regular ovarian function, but in those who cannot lose weight or if this does not work, the ovaries can be kick-started into action either using medication or by the surgical technique called ovarian drilling.

Please see Infertility in the A–Z of Symptoms chapter for more information.

Recurrent Miscarriage

The incidence of early pregnancy loss is increased in women with PCOS. Of women with recurrent miscarriage, more than 80 per cent have been identified as having polycystic ovaries. This is thought to be associated with an elevation in the serum LH (amount of luteinizing hormone in the bloodstream), as discussed previously. Also, those women who are overweight have a higher incidence of miscarriage. Weight loss has been demonstrated to help those overweight women who suffer recurrent pregnancy loss.

Diabetes in Pregnancy

The increased incidence of hyperinsulinaemia and insulin resistance means that any additional workload put on the pancreas, as occurs during any pregnancy, will make it more likely that a women will develop diabetes. If this occurs in pregnancy it is called gestational diabetes.

This may be managed by dietary modification alone, although some women will require treatment with insulin. After the pregnancy the diabetes commonly resolves, but then as we age it may reappear again in later life again (see below). The development of gestational diabetes is also associated with more complications during pregnancy.

Non-insulin-dependent Diabetes

A woman with PCOS is 7 times more likely to develop diabetes during her lifetime than the rest of the population.[6] Following a healthy eating plan and exercising regularly can help to prevent this risk developing.

Cardiovascular Disease

Using the risk factors for cardiovascular disease which have been identified in women with PCOS, it is estimated that they have a 7-fold increased risk of having a heart attack when compared to the general population.[7,8]

Endometrial Cancer

There is little direct evidence of a link between PCOS and endometrial cancer. However, we do know that this cancer is oestrogen-driven. Unopposed oestrogen treatment will result in the development of endometrial overgrowth and, eventually for some, cancer. We know that 90 per cent of women with irregular periods who are not ovulating have polycystic ovaries. For these women their wombs will receive a continual oestrogen drive with no opposition from progesterone, which is only produced after ovulation. This continual, unopposed oestrogen drive is thought to be associated with an increased risk of this cancer and could then also be associated with an increased risk of breast cancer.

We know that endometrial cancer is closely correlated with obesity and particularly with a high dietary fat intake. The high dietary fat intake is in turn associated with an increased serum oestrogen level.

Endometriosis

PCO affects about 1 in 5 of the population; endometriosis is also very common. Hence it is not uncommon to see the two conditions in the same woman. Is there a link between the two problems?

There is no definite answer to this question, but endometriosis is a disorder where tissue similar to the lining of the womb grows at other sites in the body outside the womb – commonly in the pelvis, on the ovary and in the bowel, but also in rare sites such as the lung, eye, thigh and arm. We do not know the cause of this aberrant growth, however it is very oestrogen-dependent.

The condition may improve for some women during pregnancy, when progesterone predominates and there are no periods. Medical treatments involve creating a state of 'pseudo-pregnancy' or menopause; surgical treatment can involve removing the ovaries. Since women with PCOS and irregular periods are exposed to a prolonged oestrogen drive and (in anovular cycles) little or no progesterone production, this may make the situation for women who also have endometriosis worse.

For both groups of women, avoiding environmental pollution containing the general hormone antagonists is beneficial. (For more information about endometriosis, see the Useful Addresses chapter.)

YOUR QUESTIONS ANSWERED

✢ *Will taking the Pill to manage my PCOS have any long-term health implications?*
The long-term use of the Pill is a complicated issue and needs to be
assessed on an individual basis, balancing all the potential risks and
benefits. This needs to be addressed with a doctor who ideally has an
interest in PCOS and the issues it brings up. My personal feeling as a
doctor is that I prefer not to use it if possible just for symptom control,
especially when additional lifestyle issues have never even been given
a chance. If it offers the best alternative for contraception, this is then a
different issue. In the long term it would seem to be driving the process
in an undesirable direction. The use of the Pill appears to make the user
gradually more insulin-resistant over a period of time. As we have
discussed, increasing insulin resistance and the associated
hyperinsulinaemia will gradually made symptoms worse. This may be
why women who use the Pill for symptom relief often initially get very
good results, but then after a year or so their symptoms return. However, it
is important to have a regular period for the long-term health of the uterus.
The ways of achieving this need to be addressed for each individual.

7

Getting a Diagnosis

Finding out from your doctor whether you definitely have PCOS is the first step towards tackling the problem. However, because women with PCOS can have such differing symptoms with varying degrees of severity, it is not always immediately clear whether a woman has PCOS or another problem such as PMS or a thyroid condition.

So what can you do to help your doctor diagnose your problem correctly? And what can you expect from your doctor in return?

BEFORE YOUR APPOINTMENT

Many people turn up to see their doctor because they feel generally unwell, but cannot effectively describe what their symptoms are. Spend some time – perhaps a week or a month – noting down what you feel and when you feel it, so that you can give your doctor some concrete information and answers.

Keep a symptom diary every day, noting down how you feel both physically and emotionally.

At the same time, gather information. If you see an article or hear something on the radio which matches up with what you have been feeling, tear it out or note it down to take to your appointment.

Write down any questions you have before you go in – this will stop you forgetting to ask something you have wondered about and will also show your doctor that you feel the problem is serious.

Most importantly, believe in yourself. Don't push your worries to one side and convince yourself you are making a fuss. You are going to your doctor because you feel unwell or are concerned about your health. This is a positive action.

It is also important to get support. If you know you feel nervous around your doctor, ask a friend, partner or family member to come with you. A reasonable doctor should not query this.

Confidence Boosters

Many people feel afraid of their doctors, or as if they are wasting their time. If you are one of those that do, try these simple confidence boosters:

❈ Talking things over with friends and family can help you get your mind clear before you go into your appointment.
❈ The Bach Flower Remedy larch can help to boost confidence.
❈ Deep breathing: When you feel stress taking over, simply close your eyes and take two or three deep breaths to release the tensions you're carrying.
❈ Stress saps confidence. If you know you've got a hard day ahead, try dabbing three to four drops of soothing lavender or vetivert essential oils on to a tissue and carrying it in your pocket – take a quick whiff every time you feel tensions rising.

❈ Lower your feelings of stress in the doctor's waiting room with visualization. Close your eyes, breathe deeply and imagine yourself in beautiful, stress-free surroundings – perhaps in your ideal holiday destination. Focus on each sense in turn, imagining perhaps the feel of the sun on your skin, the sound of the waves lapping up to the beach, the smell of suntan lotion or the tang of sea breezes, the taste of a beach picnic.

AT YOUR APPOINTMENT

Explain how you feel – use your symptom diary to help you out.

Suggest that you feel you could have PCOS. If your doctor agrees that this is a possibility, ask if they will carry out tests to find out if that is the case. If your doctor does not agree, ask what other conditions or causes there might be for your symptoms. You are also entitled to a second opinion, and most doctors will be happy to refer you for a scan.

Don't forget to go through your pre-prepared list of questions. While doctors are busy people, your time is just as valuable, and you deserve to leave with the feeling that at last someone has really listened to you and that you are on the way to finding out what is wrong and have taken the first steps towards treatment options.

TESTS FOR PCOS

Your doctor can send you for an ultrasound scan and/or a blood test to determine whether you have PCOS.

Ultrasound

Ultrasound works by bouncing sound waves off your ovaries to build up a picture of their surface.

It can be used to see whether or not your ovaries have the tell-tale sign of a string of many small cysts around the edge, indicating the polycystic ovarian structure.

You will either be scanned externally over your abdomen in the way you may have seen pregnant women being scanned, or with an internal probe inserted into your vagina.

If you are being scanned externally you will be asked to drink about 1 to 2 litres of water before you go in for your scan and to resist going to the toilet, as a full bladder makes the reading clearer. An internal ultrasound does not require a full bladder.

Blood Tests

Together with an ultrasound scan, most doctors will arrange for you to have a blood test. Blood will normally be taken about 8–10 days after your next period. Obviously, if your periods are now very erratic or have stopped you will not need to wait to time the test in this way and it will be taken immediately. A number of tests or measurements will commonly be made on the blood sample. These tests will help exclude other causes of similar symptoms and confirm your diagnosis of PCOS.

Full Blood Count

This is performed to confirm that you are not anaemic. Anaemia occurs when your body cannot make sufficient red blood cells. The red blood cells carry oxygen around your body; when there are too few you can feel tired, have poor stamina and concentration, feel depressed and have a reduced libido. It does not account for any of the classic symptoms, but PCOS does not always present classically.

Thyroid Function

Either depressed or elevated thyroid activity can present with a very similar symptom pattern to PCOS. It is always important to exclude this when making the diagnosis of PCOS.

Testosterone Level

An elevated testosterone is the commonest abnormal blood test seen in women with PCOS and is responsible for many of the symptoms experienced. However, not all women with PCOS will have an abnormal level, so a normal result does not exclude the diagnosis of PCOS. This is because there is a range of normal testosterone levels and we are all different. What is a 'normal' level for one woman may cause problems in another. This is probably because most of your testosterone is carried around in the blood by a carrier protein called sex hormone binding globulin (SHBG). The more SHBG you have, the more testosterone is bound to it and the less free testosterone there is present to bind to the receptors: in the skin to cause acne, at the hair follicle to cause extra body and facial hair growth, and in the ovary where it seems to affect the normal development of the follicles and cause irregular ovulation and periods.

To assess the amount of free testosterone, the level of SHBG can also be measured.

SHBG Levels and the Free Testosterone Index

By measuring SHBG as well as the total testosterone level it is possible to calculate the free testosterone index:

Testosterone = free testosterone index/SHBG

Luteinizing Hormone (LH)

The other common biochemical abnormality is an elevation of LH. This hormone is produced by the pituitary gland in the base of the brain. One of its roles is to encourage the ovary to make testosterone. Again, by no means do all women with PCOS have an elevation of LH, so a normal level does not exclude the diagnosis.

The other gonadotrophin hormone made by the pituitary, follicle stimulating hormone (FSH), is normally measured at the same time and this tends to be normal, or slightly reduced, in women who may have PCOS.

Some doctors still like to use the ratio of FSH:LH as an indicator of PCOS. In the normal ratio when the blood is taken between days 8 and 10 of the menstrual cycle, FSH is greater than LH. For many women with PCOS this ratio is reversed and strongly suggestive of the diagnosis.

Oral Glucose Tolerance Test with Insulin Measurements

This test is the same test performed to check that a person is not developing diabetes. However, before the onset of diabetes there can be mild abnormalities, where although the glucose levels are normal during the test the insulin levels are higher than normal. This suggests a degree of hyperinsulinaemia, which simply put means too much insulin production.

The production of too much insulin in response to eating some glucose or carbohydrate is also significant in the development of symptoms for women with PCOS and longer-term health risks.

FINDING OUT ABOUT TREATMENT

Don't be afraid to ask why your doctor is prescribing a particular medication for you.

❈ Ask what that medication will do inside your body to try and help you understand why it's important to take it as prescribed.
❈ Push for choice. Don't just accept the first prescription or suggestion your doctor gives you. Ask if there are any other options, and if so, could they be better for you and your lifestyle.
❈ Drug-free treatment. If you want to try and deal with your condition without drugs, and your doctor suggests losing weight, ask if you can be referred to see a specialist dietitian or nutritionist for help.
❈ Ask for information. If you are finding the explanation from your doctor difficult to understand, ask if there are any leaflets you can take away with you, or if your doctor can refer you to a self-help organization. Sometimes talking to others who have been through a

similar problem can help you understand what is going on and make you feel clearer about what course of action you would like to take. There are few real right or wrongs, there are a number of choices and different paths you can take. You need to find a path with which you are comfortable.

Getting a Second Opinion

If you are really unhappy with the way your doctor has responded, then you can try and get a second opinion.

✤ If you are at a practice where there are several doctors, you can always make another appointment with a different doctor and say you have come back because your symptoms are persisting.

✤ Ask for a referral to a specialist such as a gynaecologist, dermatologist or endocrinologist.

✤ In the UK no doctor is obliged to refer you to a gynaecologist for a second opinion on the NHS. If you are unhappy with how things are, explain why you feel it is necessary, for example that there is a family history of gynaecological problems or that the symptoms have just got worse despite the doctor's suggestions. Also, for readers in the UK, there is always the option of going private.

If you decide to go for a second opinion it is a good idea to take someone with you. Often you will receive a lot of information, and another pair of eyes and ears can help you remember and go through all that was discussed.

YOUR QUESTIONS ANSWERED

Is there a cure?
There is no 'cure' for PCO/S because it is now believed that some women are born with a genetic predisposition or susceptibility for the condition. This susceptibility is passed down from parents to their children in their

genes. However, keeping the symptoms under control is within every woman's grasp.

Will I ever have children?
Being diagnosed with PCOS does not mean you are infertile. Most women with PCOS conceive without any problems; some women find it a little harder to get pregnant but manage without medical intervention; others find they need the help of fertility treatment, whether drug-based or just by using nutritional or natural therapies. Of course there is no guarantee, but there is plenty of help and support available if problems do occur. See the section on Fertility in the A–Z of Symptoms chapter, and the contact details in the Useful Addresses chapter to find out more.

If I do have children will I pass it on?
More than one gene is involved, so it is not possible at present to give the odds of passing PCOS on. However, many studies have found that about 50–60 per cent of the children of affected parents are also affected.

Is it my fault?
Certainly not. This would be like suggesting it is your fault for being 5 foot 10 inches tall, or having green eyes. However, recognizing your own genetic predisposition does mean that you have a choice. You can now start to take control of your life by making a number of positive lifestyle changes that will allow you to greatly help yourself, control your symptoms and improve the quality of your life, both in the short term and as you get older.

8

What Your Practitioner Can Do to Help

YOUR DOCTOR

Traditional medical treatments for PCOS have focused on relieving the symptoms that each individual woman develops. The first question that a doctor will probably ask is whether or not you are trying to get pregnant. The reason why this is such an important question is that the treatment of many of the symptoms associated with PCOS uses drugs that will not allow you to conceive at the same time.

The treatments can be broken into four main categories:

1   treatment of irregular periods
2   treatment of androgen excess (hirsutism and acne, for example)
3   treatment of anovulatory infertility
4   treatment of obesity.

Treatment of Irregular Periods

The mainstay of treatment of irregular periods has been the combined oral contraceptive pill, which is not helpful if you are trying for a baby.

This treatment takes over the control of the menstrual cycle by over-riding the production of a woman's own hormones. It also acts to increase the levels of sex hormone binding globulin (SHBG), while decreasing the ovaries' production of testosterone. This reduces the free testosterone levels and will commonly result in a reduction of androgen-dependent symptoms like acne and hirsutism, as well as regulating the cycle.

The problem with the Pill is that it exacerbates insulin resistance, which may make the symptoms worse, particularly if you want to come off the Pill at a later date. This exacerbation may also make it unsuitable for women who are already overweight.

Treatment of Androgen Excess

Excess hair (hirsutism) and acne are treated using drugs that have been shown to have an anti-androgen action. The two commonly prescribed drugs are cyproterone acetate and spironolactone. They work by stopping the binding of the activated testosterone molecule to the receptors in the skin and hair follicles. The effects take two or three months to appear and are lost soon after stopping the treatment. Both drugs may actually make irregular periods worse and are not suitable to be taken while trying to conceive. Cyproterone acetate is available in a combined oral contraceptive form called Diannette.

THE PILL: YOUR QUESTIONS ANSWERED

It was only when I came off the Pill that my PCOS developed – doesn't the Pill cause the problem?
This is a very common question. A young girl either has slightly irregular periods and her mother takes her to her doctor, who starts her on the Pill to 'regulate' her periods, or a young woman whose periods are regular uses the Pill for contraception. When these women come off the Pill their PCOS symptoms seem to start – possibly they do not have a period for a long time and gradually they may develop excess body hair.

As we have seen, the Pill is used to regulate the menstrual cycle, often as a first line of attack, without considering other possibilities. As we all tend to put on weight as we get older, this weight gain can be sufficient to expose the underlying presence of PCO, resulting in the development of symptoms.

Some of the medical community are becoming increasingly concerned since the Pill has been demonstrated to make those who take it more insulin resistant. This is not then just allowing the natural passage of time and the exposure of something that was destined to happen; the Pill's use could actually be contributing to the problem.

The Pill remains a good form of contraception, but possibly it would be sensible to look at modulating lifestyle as a first line of treatment for irregular periods (and signs of androgen excess) before resorting to the Pill, which after its use may mean that the problems, both in the short and longer term, are worse than they otherwise would have been.

Will the effectiveness of the Pill wear off after a few years?
Certainly some women who have used the Pill to control symptoms such as androgen excess find that this improvement can wear off after a number of years. This might be because as the Pill drives those who are sensitive to becoming more insulin resistant this then exacerbates their symptoms again, when initially, because the Pill results in a decrease of testosterone production, their symptoms seemed to improve.

Will I be at risk of blood clots and high blood pressure with the Pill?
All women who use the Pill are at a small but higher risk of developing a blood clot, most commonly in the leg, called a deep venous thrombosis. There is no data to separate out Pill users who have PCO from those who do not, so we cannot accurately answer this question. But those who become overweight do increase their risk of both PCO and venous thrombosis. So for women with PCOS who have a weight problem, we would have to conclude that they do have a higher risk. It must be remembered that these risks are still small, in the order of 7/100,000. The doubling of risk seen in some newer types of Pill, regardless of the presence of PCO, only takes this to 15/100,000.

Will the Pill make me put on weight? And if so, will this not make my symptoms worse?

The Pill does tend to make women put on weight. It also makes them more insulin resistant. Whether it is the weight gain that makes them insulin resistant or the increased insulin resistance that causes them to put on weight is not clear. They both occur and both are associated independently with a worsening of symptoms.

How long could I stay on the Pill before I should come off it?

The Pill can be used for a number of reasons. The length of time of use will depend on these reasons, so there is no simple answer. It will vary from individual to individual. For contraception there is data to suggest that the Pill can be used into a woman's forties. However, for women with PCO we feel that this needs to be discussed carefully with their doctor as there are a number of other issues that are important.

Treatment of Anovulatory Infertility

For those wishing to conceive there are essentially three strategies. The other symptoms tend to be ignored while these treatments are tried, since the treatments mentioned either stop conception occurring or are not safe to be taken while pregnant.

To stimulate the ovaries to ovulate again and allow the return of a regular cycle, clomiphene citrate is often the first line of therapy. This drug works by inhibiting the feedback of oestrogen to the pituitary. The pituitary then increases the production of follicle stimulating hormone (FSH) to try to raise the levels of oestrogen. This results in more follicles being developed. A consequence of this is that twins and triplet pregnancies are more common. Recent recommendations suggest that clomiphene should not be given for more than six cycles, as prolonged use may increase the risk of developing ovarian cancer in later life.

For those in whom clomiphene does not work, doctors now go on to use injections of FSH directly. These injections must be given into the skin daily, in the same way as some people with diabetes give themselves insulin injections. The follicle development must be monitored carefully using ultrasound scans every other day to ensure no more than two follicles are ever released at one time. This injection program has proved very successful, although it is intensive for both patient and doctor.

As an alternative to this, or if this is not successful, some patients will move on to assisted conception techniques such as in vitro fertilization (IVF).

An alternative to these medical treatments includes laser or electro-cautery to the ovary, in a process known as ovarian drilling. In these techniques a number of the cysts within the ovary are destroyed. This seems to allow ovulation to re-establish its sensitivity to the pituitary's production of FSH and begin to ovulate again. This procedure has fallen in and out of favour. It is often seen as a last resort and is not used in all treatment centres. It can be very difficult to carry out in overweight patients, and its effects are short lived – normally six months to one year.

Treatment of Obesity

Weight management of patients with PCOS by doctors has often not been successful. This may be because of the techniques employed, although there are certainly some notable exceptions. Even relatively small reductions in body weight appear to have a large effect on reproductive function.

Over the last few years there have been a number of preparations that inhibit the absorption of fat from the diet. Several of these have been shown to be useful in weight-reduction programs. However they are not selective in what fats they inhibit the absorption of. Because of our need for essential fats, particularly in pregnancy when they are used to form the baby's brain, these preparations cannot be recommended. See the sensible four-point plan (from page 100), which will encourage safe and long-term weight loss.

Lowering Insulin Resistance

Reports have appeared in the scientific literature on the treatment of insulin resistance seen in PCOS using insulin-sensitizing agents. Metformin, a treatment often used to treat non-insulin-dependent diabetes, has been found to have uses in treating all of the classic symptoms of PCOS. It reduces insulin, testosterone and luteinizing hormone (LH) levels and appears to increase the levels of sex hormone binding globulin (SHBG). These biochemical changes have been associated with a return to a regular menstrual cycle, ovulation, weight loss and a reduction in the symptoms of androgen excess. It seems to counter all the unwanted effects of having PCO/S, so is it the answer?

Well, it has all the same effects as a healthy lifestyle, as we will see later. It could be seen as a help to those who are not able to help themselves, and so will undoubtedly find a place in the doctor's armoury. However, all medications that offer benefits also have side-effects and contra-indications. The list of current contra-indications for Metformin includes endocrine disorders, infections, pregnancy, lactation and stress. This is possibly because many of these areas have yet to be researched adequately. Hopefully this work will be forthcoming. However, good lifestyle management is simple, safe and cost effective and possibly should be the first line of attack rather than resorting to a drug treatment.

For more help, support and information if you are trying to get pregnant, see Fertility and Pre-conceptual Care in the Useful Addresses chapter.

COMPLEMENTARY THERAPIES

Any qualified complementary practitioner treats the whole person as an individual, so will tailor-make a prescription after building up a detailed picture of the person's whole health – looking at the ways in which a hormonal imbalance is displayed in that person and looking at the reasons why it may be happening, such as the drugs they have taken or are taking, their lifestyle, including diet and exercise, and their emotional well-being including emotional difficulties such as depression and low self-esteem, which may occur as a result of PCOS. The practitioner will also look at outside stresses such as your job, finances and family issues.

In order to build up this picture effectively, a first appointment with a complementary practitioner often lasts an hour to an hour and a half. You should take this as an opportunity to ask about what realistic improvements the therapist feels they can achieve with your help. This prevents you from expecting too much and then being disappointed. It also helps you to assess whether you want to carry on with the treatment.

The cost of complementary treatments can be a barrier, but bear in mind that some therapists ask for payment on a sliding scale according to your income, and give discounted treatments to students and the unwaged. Your doctor can also refer you to a complementary therapist on the NHS in the UK. You may get cheaper treatments by having your session with a trainee therapist who is overseen by a qualified practitioner. For details of these cheaper therapy options consult the governing bodies listed in the Useful Addresses chapter.

In the same way that good doctors who find themselves out of their depth will often refer you to see a specialist, a complementary practitioner who feels you need extra support, perhaps emotionally, may suggest that you think about seeking help through counselling or by joining a support group. They may also suggest that you take up a relaxation or stress-management program, whether by joining a local yoga or meditation class, booking yourself in for a relaxing treatment such as massage, shiatsu or healing, or just making sure you organize some time for yourself in your daily schedule.

Many of these therapies are also very relaxing, and the combination of the therapeutic benefits, the relaxation and the sense of emotional release from talking about your problem and giving yourself some time to focus on what you need can all combine to bring about a powerful healing experience.

Trying over-the-counter remedies is no substitute for seeing a practitioner who can assess your own particular needs, provide an individually tailored prescription and oversee your progress. Some, but not all, complementary therapists are happy to treat women taking the Pill, and many are happy to help treat a woman going through the emotional and physical process of fertility treatment, but you should ask about this before making an appointment or when you first see a practitioner.

If you would like to consult a qualified practitioner in any complementary discipline, or find out more about it, see the Useful Addresses chapter.

Featured here are the complementary therapies which women with PCOS seem to finding most helpful in dealing with their symptoms. The evidence is anecdotal and comes from talking to women with PCOS about how they are managing their condition.

Getting the Most from Your Treatment

❋ Choose a therapy with which you will feel comfortable – for example, if you don't like needles, acupuncture would not be a good bet, and if you feel self-conscious about your body, massage may be something you would like to try only as your confidence builds, rather than at the beginning.

❋ Vegetarians need to check with therapies such as homoeopathy, nutritional therapy and Traditional Chinese Medicine that the remedies they are taking contain no animal ingredients.

❋ Liking and trusting your therapist is incredibly important – many patients don't take the medication prescribed to them by a doctor whose attitude or methods they don't like, because they don't feel hopeful or motivated after their visit. You must make sure that you feel comfortable with your therapist before investing in a course of treatment, as this could affect how well you respond and how much effort you put into making any lifestyle changes they may suggest.

❀ Make sure the therapist you see is qualified and reputable by approaching the governing bodies and national institutions (see Useful Addresses) associated with the therapy. Some complementary therapists work together with doctors, and doctors will refer patients to them. This is obviously a good sign.

Acupuncture

Women with PCOS seem to have found acupuncture most helpful for kickstarting non-existent periods and for regulating lengthy cycles. Maria Mercati, acupuncturist and Chinese massage therapist who has set up the BodyHarmonics Centre in Cheltenham, England, says Traditional Chinese Medicine would seek to address the pattern of Qi disharmony that underlies the hormonal dysfunction in PCOS. Qi (also sometimes known as *chi*) is the vital energy of the body, which helps to keep it healthy and full of vitality. Qi runs through the body in channels known as meridians, each of which corresponds to different areas and organs of the body. In Chinese theory, it is blockages in this energy flow which cause stagnation of the Qi energy, and ill-health.

The diagnosis would take into account all the varying symptoms of PCOS and how they manifest in the individual who has come for a treatment. An acupuncturist would commonly work on liver Qi and spleen Qi deficiency for abnormal bleeding, and possibly kidney Qi imbalance, but specific needling points would be determined by the individual case and indications from Chinese pulse and tongue examinations.

Treatment would normally be daily, starting from around day 21 of your period and until your period starts, then repeated each month until the condition improves.

A needling prescription would be tailored to the individual, but for PCOS you should expect to have needles placed in points in the abdomen as well as the arms and legs. The patient should not experience pain but does need to feel some sensation as part of the therapy and this could be uncomfortable.

Aromatherapy

Aromatherapy has been cited as both a relaxing and therapeutic therapy, which uses the aromatic essential oils from plants, flowers, trees and fruits as the active ingredients in treatment. Suitable oils are selected based on the patient's emotional and physical situation and the symptoms she exhibits.

The oils can be administered through the skin in a massage (they are absorbed into the bloodstream effectively this way – think of HRT and nicotine patches, which also demonstrate that the skin is a useful way to deliver treatment), or through the blood vessels in the lining of the nose by inhalation, when the oils are put on a diffuser or burner.

Aromatherapist Frances Box, who specializes in fertility issues including PCOS, uses aromatherapy along with reflexology at Ceres Natural Health and Beauty in Sussex and Surrey in the UK, says she chooses aromatherapy oils both to help regulate the hormonal imbalances in PCOS and to aid relaxation and the release of emotional stress, which she feels are great contributors towards ill-health. An aromatherapist could use the following oils during your treatment:

❋ For hormonal balance: Vitex agnus castus (see page 95), geranium and rose
❋ For relaxation: sandalwood, neroli, ylang ylang and mandarin

Shirley Price Aromatherapy also suggests that the relaxing and anti-inflammatory properties of camomile would be helpful.

Homoeopathy

Homoeopaths will build up a complex picture of a person's health and emotional history in the same way as other complementary therapists. This allows them to use what are known as constitutional remedies, which can be selected to match your homoeopathic constitution, something determined by your health history and your emotional attitude to life.

Constitutional remedies work at a deep level to try and encourage your body and mind to shift from current negative patterns into more positive ones.

Homoeopath Moira Houston has worked with many women with PCOS. She says that specific remedies to target individual symptoms can be used along with general constitutional remedies. For example, a remedy called silica could be used to help with acne.

You would take the constitutional remedy once, but would probably need to take the specific symptom remedies twice a day – they are usually given in the form of small white pillules. You would come back to assess the effects in a month to six weeks, and keep coming back to monitor improvements. Moira says it usually takes around a month or two for a woman to feel better in herself and have more energy, though menstrual regulation may take six months or more and perhaps need lifestyle changes and a close look at emotional attitudes towards being a woman in order to feel more positive and help the treatment be most effective.

Medical Herbalism

Anecdotally, among women with PCOS medical herbalism is perhaps the most popular and effective alternative therapy for getting to grips with the condition and its many and various symptoms, as well as providing support for a smooth transition if a woman decides to stop taking the contraceptive Pill.

As mentioned above, each herbal treatment is unique, but if you visit a practitioner these are some of the herbs whose names you may come across, says Medical Herbalist Fiona Waller, who has great experience of treating PCOS. (Please note that this is not intended as a guide for self-medication.)

❋ to encourage hormonal balance: Vitex agnus castus (chaste tree – see page 95), false unicorn root, sarsaparilla (containing steroid-like substances which has a progesterogenic action in the body), the

Chinese remedy white paeony (which has been shown to counter high androgen levels in women with PCOS when combined with liquorice)

✻ tonics to the reproductive system: Chinese angelica/Dong quai, blue cohosh and motherwort, among many others

✻ to aid the liver in metabolizing hormones and encourage efficient excretion via the bowel: Marigold, milk thistle and rosemary, among many

✻ for stress and emotional issues: German chamomile, lavender, St John's Wort, vervain and lemon balm, among many others

✻ for skin problems (in addition to hormone balancers and those to aid the liver and digestion): immune-boosting echinacea, purifying nettle

Dr Ann Walker, a medical herbalist, nutritionist and research scientist based at the University of Reading's Hugh Sinclair Unit of Human Nutrition, also explains that many herbalists will suggest beneficial changes to diet and lifestyle as the basis for good health, and use herbal medicines as an additional resource for helping you back on the way to good health. She also stresses that herbalism can be used as a support for a woman with PCOS to help deal with symptoms such as acne or irregular periods while she undertakes longer-term diet and lifestyle changes.

Nutritional Therapy

Good nutrition is the mainstay of all good health; without it, sooner or later you will become unwell. As we have seen, what, when and how you eat may all affect the symptoms and course of the problems experienced by women who suffer with PCOS.

Many of our dietary habits are cultural or driven by fashion or the pressure of our hectic lives. Looking at and considering what you may need to change means not only assessing what you are currently eating, but getting a full medical and social history to reflect your individual needs. Everyone is unique. Each person's genetic make-up, age, sex, medical history, exposure to pollution, previous diets and ability to digest and absorb nutrients will be distinctive. In addition, nutritional needs are not static; they change with advancing years, stress levels, exercise regimes and overall health.

A good nutritional therapist will offer an assessment of your current situation, design a management plan for change (because it is not possible nor desirable to make too many changes at once), monitor your progress over a set time scale and modulate your program as you make progress, dealing with any new issues that develop. The process should involve a detailed history and examination followed by a discussion of the changes that are required. As in any medical setting, any investigations should be appropriate and explained fully. The first consultation usually takes 1 hour; thereafter the number of consultations and their length will depend on the amount of work that is needed and the support required to effect this work.

Matt Lovell, a clinical nutritionist at the Centre of Nutritional Medicine, explains that typically you will need to take supplements to support you while you are making diet and lifestyle changes. The work should be focused very much on the changes you need to make; once they have been made it is usually possible to reduce the number of supplements you are taking, or stop taking them altogether.

Reflexology

Many women with PCOS have found reflexology helpful, saying it relaxes them and helps their cycle become more regular.

This treatment feels like a vigorous foot massage, during which a practitioner stimulates specific reflex points on the foot which are thought to link into energy channels called meridians running throughout the body, as in Chinese medicine. By pressing one reflex point in the foot, the therapist influences the energy flow around all the other organs and body areas which run along that meridian.

Qualified reflexologist and aromatherapist Frances Box, who specializes in fertility issues, says that a reflexologist treating PCOS would often focus on the reflex point for the pituitary gland in order to influence hormonal balance, as well as perhaps working on the points for the ovary and other points for general well-being and relaxation.

Vitex Agnus Castus – The Women's Herb

Vitex agnus castus (also known as chaste tree and monk's pepper) has been used for women's health and hormonal problems for over 2,500 years. First mentioned in Homer's Iliad in the 6th century BC, it was one of the medicinal plants officially recognized in the ancient world, being recommended by the Greek physician Hippocrates for stopping bleeding after labour, and by Roman physician Pliny (AD 23–79) for promoting menstruation.

Dried berries of the shrub are used mainly to treat menstrual problems, particularly in Germany, where Vitex was rediscovered in the 1930s and is now prescribed by doctors in a liquid form called Agnolyt to help regulate hormone levels.

Research into Vitex has been going on for more than 30 years, and has proved to be of significant help for women with PMS, reducing physical and psychological symptoms such as breast pain, headaches, cravings, increased appetite and mood swings.

Vitex can also increase milk production in breastfeeding women, though it should not be used during pregnancy.

Because Vitex stimulates the production of the hormone progesterone, it was initially thought to be a 'natural HRT' with a direct hormonal action. Studies in the 1940s and 1950s showed that it does not, in fact, contain hormones, though it does work on the pituitary gland, which produces hormones. It increases the amount of luteinizing hormone (LH) released by the pituitary gland, and the result is a balance of the progesterone and oestrogen produced by the ovaries during the menstrual cycle. This can have effects beyond normalizing the menstrual cycle – progesterone is essential to pregnancy, for example, as its presence is necessary for a fertilized egg to establish itself in the uterus, and it also contributes to milk production.

Vitex is classified as adaptogenic (i.e., it adapts to the specific needs of the body). So on the one hand it can treat PMS and menopausal symptoms (thought to be caused by over-production of oestrogen); and on the other, post-menopausal problems (caused by under-production of oestrogen).

Capsules and tinctures are derived from the whole dried berry. Their different components (oils, flavonoids, iridoids) have not yet been tested separately, though all of them are thought to be medicinally active.

A 1997 survey at the University of Reading has shown that, among members of the National Institute of Medical Herbalists in Britain, Vitex is principally used in the treatment of hormonal problems such as PMS or post-menopausal problems. There have been no clinical studies on the effects of Vitex on menopausal symptoms, but some users say it is comparable to HRT (synthetic hormones) in helping with symptoms like fluid retention and depression.

In the survey, 80 per cent of respondents used it to treat female acne, and 90 per cent used it for female infertility – possible only in cases where infertility is caused by a menstrual cycle disorder. In 1988 a trial involving 48 women who had infertility associated with hormone levels produced positive results: 25 achieved normal levels of progesterone after taking Vitex, and 15 of them became pregnant.

9

Helping Yourself

Discovering that you have PCOS can be a shock. It can also be a relief, because you finally know why you have been having health problems. Once you have come to terms with the fact that you have PCOS, the next step is doing something about it. Your doctor can help you to do this, as can a qualified complementary health practitioner. But one of the most satisfying ways to face your condition in a positive frame of mind is to try and help yourself.

Many people who are diagnosed with an illness or condition of some sort say that they feel frustrated that medical professionals seem to take over once a diagnosis has been made, and allow them little input into their recovery. The psychological benefits of doing something for yourself are hard to beat.

PCOS might be a chronic condition, but that doesn't mean you have to put up with it interfering in your life. There is a lot you can do to help yourself.

Earlier chapters have explained where PCOS is thought to come from genetically, and the factors such as diet, exercise, stress and pollution which can help to bring on the symptoms or make them worse. There's nothing you can do to change your genetic make-up, but you can do an awful lot to change your lifestyle.

This is a big commitment. Changing the foods you eat, building exercise into your routine when you may feel tired and self-conscious, and trying to cut out the amount of environmental toxins you absorb is going to be a slow process. And you can't just try on these changes for a few weeks and then go back to old habits. Eating right and living well are long-term goals to help you live the rest of your life feeling the best you can feel even if you do have PCOS.

These changes are aimed at getting right to the heart of the deep-down problems that cause PCOS, rather than simply treating the symptoms that appear as a result of them. But getting to the root of the problem takes time, patience and effort.

Being realistic about making these changes to your life is one of the most important things you can do. There is no point setting yourself impossible goals and targets; you will only make yourself miserable when you don't reach them. While the plan outlined here advises healthy eating and exercise, don't get angry with yourself if you end up eating the odd piece of cake or treating yourself to a big greasy burger and fries. See it as a special occasion, enjoy it and move on.

You must also bear in mind that you are not being persecuted simply because you have PCOS, so don't feel resentment towards your condition and blame it or your body for depriving you. Eating more and more healthy food and cutting down on processed, foods, fat and sugar are basic ways to help yourself feel healthier whether you have an illness or not. It's just that these changes will make more of a difference to you if you happen to have PCOS.

The self-help management plan in the next chapter is designed to help you implement practical changes in your day-to-day life that will make a difference to how you feel. But it could be 3, 6 or even 12 months before you really start to notice a big difference in how your symptoms start to come under control. Having said this, you may notice that some symptoms disappear or lessen much more quickly than others.

Being committed and patient is hard work, and if there aren't any instant results it is tempting to give up. But the good news is that you can do plenty in the mean time to help deal with your particular symptoms, to give you a quick boost while you are carrying out the long-term changes in the background. The A–Z of Symptoms and self-help tips you can use to deal with them follow the long-term management plan outlined in the next chapter.

Using a combined approach of the long-term plan and more immediate symptom-solving strategies will help you to feel better. And the better you feel, the more inspired you will be to carry on.

10

Four-point Management Plan

The medical management of women who have PCOS has traditionally been focused on specific symptoms. This management tends, by and large, to be drug-orientated. This is not because doctors do not recognize the benefits of lifestyle changes that might also offer the same effects. It's because getting people to make changes in the way they live their lives is just not easy. It takes education, motivation and time. Of these, doctors are normally only able to offer the first, and because it is limited by the amount of time they can devote to you, even this can be difficult to obtain.

This four-point management plan should not be seen as an alternative to standard medical practice. It is an essential partner. It will allow you to begin to take control of your life and your symptoms. You will find that most doctors are normally very supportive of patients who are prepared to help themselves. While doing this you may also find that, over a period of time, you can become less dependent on drugs to treat symptoms, and that this offers you the choice of taking less or even no medication.

It is important that the decisions to alter any medication you are currently taking should be discussed and made with your own medical practitioner. However – and possibly contrary to popular belief – the aim of medical practice is not to give patients drugs, although they represent a major part of the doctor's tool kit. Most doctors are absolutely delighted if, as a consequence of a lifestyle change, their patient no longer needs a medication. Remember, too, that most medications do have side-effects. Weight reduction can mean that a woman who previously may have required drugs to treat her high blood pressure and her diabetes no longer requires these medications and can avoid the loss of libido that one of them was causing.

Get Motivated

In the process of change, the main factor – once a problem has been recognized – is the motivation to do something about it. It can be difficult to stick to a resolution to change your lifestyle if the good effects cannot be seen immediately.

The motivation to change your lifestyle has to come from within you. It's like stopping smoking. No one else can make you do it. So give yourself some short-term goals – such as getting into a dress a size smaller, or getting rid of your acne. Bear in mind that everyone will have different goals, and what your doctor or a friend may consider to be important might be the thing that matters least to you. It's what you feel and think that counts here.

The advantage of small goals is that you will tend to get quicker results. Succeeding is very important, so there is nothing wrong with taking one small step at a time. This becomes a bit like saving – if you look after the small things today (the pennies, or in this case any day-to-day activities that could help you avoid getting acne or having to move up into that next dress size) – then the bigger things will look after themselves (the heart disease and diabetes!). So identify one or a number of small goals that will improve your life *right now*.

You Might Not Like It at First...

Most smokers tend to forget the fact that the first cigarette they smoked made them feel sick; most beer drinkers didn't like the taste when they first tried it. Nevertheless, when it comes to it they find it difficult to give up these old ingrained habits. The same is true of many changes: it may take some time before they feel comfortable or natural. But in the end you may find that you prefer water to a cola drink, or enjoy exercise as much as watching TV.

If you have ever tried to cut down on the sugar in your tea or coffee, you will know that at first the drink tastes terrible, but you soon get to the stage where you think it tastes awful with the extra sugar back in.

When you make changes they may not feel, taste, look, smell or even sound fun at the time, but based on sound sensible advice and, given some time to feel the benefits, you need never go back. You will be able to attain your goals and see an improvement in the quality of your life.

Give Yourself Time

In going through the four-point plan you may recognize many things or areas in your life that you would like to change. This recognition will no doubt be correct, but remember it is very difficult to change everything all at the same time. It would be like making fifteen New Year's resolutions all on the same New Year's Eve party. A week later you'd find you have not been able to keep up any of them. Don't set yourself up to fail. What is more, even if you are able to cope with multiple changes undertaken simultaneously it is unlikely that those around you, including family and friends, will. At home it is certainly better to have evolution rather than revolution.

To be successful, give yourself and those you live with some time. This does not mean that you should do nothing. Remember, if you are living in a family setting you will be more successful if the changes you are proposing can be adopted by everyone. You are not going on a new fad diet. You are gradually changing the way you (and possibly those around you) live.

It typically takes about three months to effect a number of the more major changes. The full benefits of these changes may take many months or even years to be seen, although even after a week or two most people will notice considerable improvements. Once the main areas have been dealt with you will find you can gradually refine and improve your plan. This should be an ongoing reappraisal, because our bodies are not static. We are all ageing, and as we age our unique requirements will gradually change – and with this our plan may need to be modified. This should be expected.

It may have taken five years to get to the position you are in at the moment, fed up with symptoms you wish you did not have, so it is likely to take some time to reverse it.

This four-point management plan will give you a good general guide to allow you to plan and start to move in the right direction to achieve your personal goals. However, everyone is unique and because of this it must be remembered that this can only be a general plan, as good as it might be. Ideally everyone should be assessed as an individual. Where possible we would recommend that you identify a local healthcare team who can offer additional specific guidance that will allow you to tailor and fine-tune this plan for your own specific needs, especially if you are considering wanting to change any medication you might be taking. Plan your changes, and remember it will take some time and consider getting some support. Besides healthcare workers, remember that an excellent place to turn to for support can be found in others who have PCOS. Verity and PCOSupport, as well as e-groups on the Internet, certainly offer this type of help. For more suggestions please see the Useful Addresses chapter.

DETOXIFICATION

We have seen how pollution can contribute towards PCOS. Reducing your exposure is a good thing to do to help yourself.

There are many published 'detox diets' recommending you drink only water and vegetable juice for a number of days, then allow you to add in other foods over a week or so. The problem with these 'diets' is that they represent a quick fix that is normally unsustainable in the longer term. If you cannot keep to them, although they may help to detoxify your system in the short term they will teach you little about how to live your life.

Your body is approximately 70 per cent water, and so water is probably the most important nutrient in your body. Without it we cannot survive, and we are only too aware that contaminated water represents a serious health risk in many parts of the world. In starting a program which commences with detoxifying, making sure the water you drink is clean and pure is a good first action.

Water, Water

The standard purification techniques used by most water companies remove the matter and bugs from the water by and large, but do not remove all the dissolved chemicals. Most water companies will test for about 50 or 60 chemicals. These include things like lead. Even today, many houses still contain old lead pipes that will produce unexpectedly high levels of lead contamination. But this is the least of the current problems. It is estimated that as many as 60,000 different chemicals now contaminate our water supplies. In the US it is suggested that all the ground water is contaminated with man-made chemicals. In attempts to clean the water, other chemicals are sometimes added, including chlorine and aluminium. Not only may these chemicals be toxic in their own right, but chlorine may react with organic wastes to form trihalomethanes. These compounds are known to increase the risk of cancer of the colon, rectum and bladder.

The recognition that much of our tap water is contaminated has been seen with the boom in bottled water manufacturers. Many of these companies, however, sell normal tap water that has simply been passed through a filter. There is also no need to drink 'mineral water' to obtain the minerals we need for our body. The main source of our minerals comes from vegetables we eat grown on mineral-rich soil. It is not possible to assimilate many inorganic minerals. They are absorbed when bound to other molecules found in normal foods.

The best source of water is distilled water or, alternatively, a multiple filter reverse-osmosis system. These systems can be fitted to the mains water system at home. They allow you to use as much water as you want, safely, without the bother of having to carry bottles home from the super-market. Any system that you buy should be able to reduce the contamination to less than 10 parts per million. That's about as clean as you can get.

If installing a system like this is too expensive or you live in rented accommodation, try buying a portable filter which uses cartridges to help get rid of chemicals such as nitrate fertilizers. Alternatively, buy glass-bottled water for drinking, or drink cooled boiled tap water – this at least helps get rid of any bacteria and reduces the amount of 'hard water' limescale you are drinking in.

Once you have a clean water supply, use it. Adults need to drink 2 to 3 litres of pure water each day. Remember that when you exercise this need will increase dramatically. Athletes in heavy training can use as much as 10 litres in one day. Becoming dehydrated during exercise will have a major impact on your performance or ability to continue and get the maximum benefit. Since everyone's time is increasingly pressured, avoid not getting the best out of yourself just because you have not drunk enough water. Even small water losses of 2–3 per cent can result in a 10 per cent reduction in strength.

What is more, your thirst reflex is a poor indicator of your state of hydration. Do not wait until you feel thirsty before you have a drink. Plan to drink regularly throughout the day. You can replace the water with any beverage, but remember that many of them will contain other chemicals like caffeine, or added sugar, which will have effects you may want to avoid. Alcoholic drinks, besides being high in refined carbohydrates, have a dehydrating effect and so will actually make any dehydration worse.

Clean Up Your Air

The amount of air pollution we breathe in is increasing, and adding another layer of polluting chemicals for our bodies to process. Help to reduce your air pollution intake with these quick tips.

- ❈ Go for a walk at lunchtime. If you work in a city, head for a park or green space, as trees give out more energizing oxygen.
- ❈ Sleep with an ionizer on. Air by the coast leaves you feeling relaxed and sleepy because it has more negative ions in it than normal. An ionizer turns positive ions in your room into negative ions, giving you an extra soothing sleep.
- ❈ Surround your work space and house with plants. NASA research has shown that the following plants can extract substances such as fumes from chemical cleaners, perfumes and aftershaves, radon and cigarette smoke from the air as well as chemicals from printers, photocopiers and VDUs: peace lilies, dwarf banana plants, spider plants, coconut palms and weeping figs. Or give yourself a happiness boost as well, with the cheerful colours of purifying chrysanthemums and gerberas.

Eating Better Food

Organic or Not, Does It Matter?
The simple answer is yes – buying organic food is better for your health. This has been confirmed by recent research from the UK Soil Association. Organically-grown foods come from farms that use farming techniques that are sustainable and support the environment. These techniques result in good quality soil that is not mineral deficient.

Crops are only as good as the soil they are grown in. Animals reared on the land are only as good as the grass and feed they get to eat. Organically-grown vegetables are more nutrient dense and obviously contain no additional chemical toxins. Organically-reared livestock, because they have to be allowed to roam to find food naturally, have meat that is considerably leaner than animals that have been intensively farmed. Intensively-farmed animals do not get to use their muscles normally, as they are often kept in very cramped, overcrowded enclosures. Their meat is fatty and they can be encouraged to put on additional fatty muscle with the use of steroids. The more meat an animal produces, the better the price in the market place.

The fat that we consume from animals is mainly saturated fat. This represents one of the types of fat we should be trying to reduce within our diets, so eating organically-grown meats reduces your saturated fat intake and avoids exposure to other non-food chemicals. So organic foods are not only more nutrient dense, those nutrients are of a better quality.

Most supermarkets now sell a great deal of organic produce, but it can be expensive. Try and buy just one item a week when you shop to get into the habit of looking at organic food as an investment in your health. You can also get boxes of seasonal fruit and vegetables delivered to your door, and there are mail order services which can provide everything from milk to mushrooms. In the US there are many organic farmers markets where farmers sell directly to the public, cutting out the middle man and cutting down the price. These have now caught on in certain parts of the UK. Try contacting local government or your neighbourhood health food store about getting local, cheaper organic foods. To find out more about buying organic food, see the Useful Addresses chapter.

If you can't afford or can't find organic foods, make sure you wash all vegetables thoroughly, in a mixture of water with a capful of organic cider vinegar or using a special product such as Veggiewash, designed to help get rid of pesticides and germs. It can also be worth peeling vegetables such as carrots, which have been found to harbour a large amount of chemical residues in their outer skins. For more information see the Healthy Eating section of the Useful Addresses chapter.

Read the Label

Many foods are processed to make them appear more enticing and 'improve' the flavour. The main aim of these techniques is actually to improve shelf-life. Fresh food goes off quite rapidly. All these post-harvest processes will further reduce the nutrient content of your food, and add non-food chemicals. In food processing many foods will also have sugar and salt added to them. We have described the effects of these additives on women with PCOS before. It is important to read the labels of any packaged food. Ninety-nine percent of fat-free foods normally have additional sugar and/or salt added, since removing the fat removes much of the taste. The sugar will be converted into triglyceride fat and stored as central body fat and laid down within the blood vessels, producing a furring of the arteries or atherosclerosis. Additional salt will tend to increase your blood pressure.

High blood pressure and increasing body fat, especially centrally (around your middle), are things to be avoided. Generally women put on weight in one of two ways: so that they resemble in body shape either an apple or a pear. What has been identified over recent years is that the people who put on their fat centrally, to give an apple-shaped body with a large tummy and thinner arms and legs, have a greater risk of developing both non-insulin-dependent diabetes and heart disease. It seem that the fat laid down in the abdomen is 'metabolically' active. What this means is that it affects the liver's insulin and fat metabolism. It seems to encourage hyperinsulinaemia and insulin resistance. This is the same type of fat deposition that is seen in Cushings syndrome when someone is exposed to too much of the adrenal stress hormone cortisol. These patients also have a greater risk of non-insulin-dependent diabetes and heart disease.

The pear-shape fat deposition does not increase these risks. It is metabolically inert. The difference is thought to be that the blood supply from central fat goes directly to the liver where it can exert an effect, whereas the blood supply from fat in the thighs has to go around the body before reaching the liver, so the effect is reduced.

Food Packaging

Many processed foods come in packets ready to warm up before eating. They are stored wrapped in plastic and aluminium. Both of these storage methods will add additional non-food chemicals into your food, and this is greatly compounded by heating. Cans of fizzy drinks contain six times the amount of aluminium compared to the same beverages in glass bottles. There is always a small amount of plastic residue that dissolves into drinks from the lining of a can or from a plastic bottle. Glass bottles are much better than plastic. Also, avoid heating food wrapped in plastic.

Be Realistic

Does all this mean you can never have unfiltered water or a non-organic carrot again? Not at all, but remember the 80:20 rule. If you can get it right 80 per cent of the time, you are doing well. You still have to live in the real world and it is no good becoming a social hermit, as this will not be beneficial in the long term. When you are at a friend's house and she offers you a plate of chips, just say 'thank you'. When you're out at dinner, choose sensibly, but don't punish yourself.

The best place to start is at home. It is your environment, so you are more likely to be able to exert control over it.

Detoxification lifestyle changes obviously take a bit of effort to organize, but it will not only benefit you it will benefit the whole family and all those you live with. Certainly children have been demonstrated to suffer less attention deficit disorder and hyper-activity when their diets are improved to eliminate non-food chemicals.

IMPROVING WHAT YOU EAT

Once you have thought about reducing your chemical overload by choosing certain types of food, it is time to consider the balance of what you eat.

To Diet or Not to Diet?

We need to spend a moment considering what exactly is meant by the word 'diet'. In truth we would very much like to strike the word from our vocabulary because it has, like many words in the English language, more than one meaning. It can be used as a term to generally describe the food that you eat, but it is also used to mean a change in the food that you eat that you hope will produce a positive effect such as weight loss.

The second use of the word refers to something that is commonly done for a short period of time, to achieve the desired effect, after which the original 'diet' is reverted to. When reverting to the old or normal diet, whatever positive effects were obtained from the new diet are then lost, and we move on towards a situation of yo-yo dieting or crash dieting. We may lurch from one 'magical' diet to the next, each with a small amount of success but which is impossible to stick to so the weight returns (often with a vengeance).

The problem is that any rapid weight loss tends to be a loss of body muscle, and not fat. So although lighter in weight, as a percentage of your body weight you are carrying more body fat and are therefore fatter than when you started. Since it is the body fat that is undesirable and also part of the cause of the metabolic problems encountered for women with PCOS, crash dieting is not only unsuccessful, but frankly dangerous.

We are not interested in a short-term diet, which you will ignore again once you feel better. We would like to encourage you to make a number of lifestyle changes to the food that you choose to eat, to allow you to continue to make long-term sustained progress in achieving your personal goals.

Ignore Calorie Counting

Calorie counting is unrealistic and doesn't take into account the fact that you could eat a chocolate bar and nothing else for a day to stick inside your calorie limit, which clearly isn't a healthy way to eat. We normally find that by just altering the type and timing of the food eaten, most people will lose a considerable amount of weight. When this is combined with a small amount of exercise, the weight loss is always pronounced and possible to maintain in the long term.

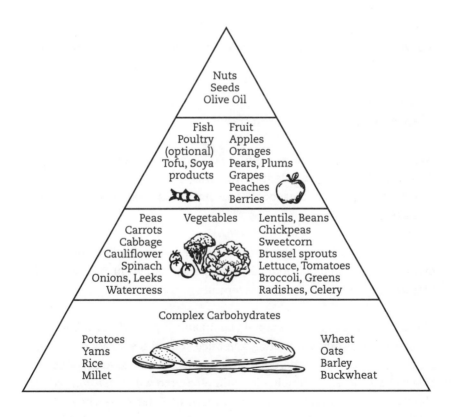

Figure 12

Basic Principles

In 1992 the US Department of Agriculture proposed the food pyramid (see Figure 12). This suggests that 30–45 per cent of your calories should come from whole grains, 15–25 per cent from vegetables, 10–15 per cent from fruit, less than 10 per cent from meat and dairy products, and no more than 5 per cent from sugar and fats.

This is very good in theory, but in practice the average Western diet consists of 37 per cent fat and 50 per cent refined carbohydrates and refined sugar. And this diet is not healthy for most people, and actually makes the symptoms of PCOS worse.

We would recommend each day you should gradually adjust your diet so that you eat:

Five portions of vegetables
Four portions of wholegrains such as rice
Three portions of fruit
Two to five portions of protein, which should include some vegetable sources such as beans, lentils and tofu
One portion (one tablespoon) of essential fats such as cold-pressed flaxseed oil.

Bear in mind that when we say fruit and vegetables this includes fresh, dried, frozen, tinned (without added sugar, salt or syrup) and also freshly pressed juice (not made from concentrate or cordial).

These fruits and vegetables should be organic if possible, avoiding processed foods and attempting to reduce your intake of added salt. As for drinks, it must be remembered that many drinks like tea, coffee and cola contain caffeine. Caffeine is a stimulant and will cause your adrenal glands to release additional stress hormones. We have seen how these may exacerbate symptoms for women suffering with PCOS. This does not mean that you should never have a coffee, but consider limiting this to no more than one caffeine drink each day.

Juicers

A very good way of getting an extra fruit and vegetable fix is to invest in a juicer and make your own freshly-pressed juices such as carrot and apple, apple and kiwi, carrot, apple and celery, apple, banana and mango, or whatever mixture takes your fancy. Drink the juice as soon as you have made it for the best benefit. The down-side to juicers is that they extract the pulp so you don't get the benefit of the fibre. If you want the fibre, try using a blender to make smoothie-type drinks using bananas, berries, soft fruits such as peaches and pears, and soya milk or organic low-fat yoghurts.

Smoking

We have not mentioned much about smoking, because we think that most people are now aware of the harm it will cause. It is a significant anti-nutrient. The simple advice is to stop. It is often quoted as the single biggest health improvement anyone can make.

And it is not only smoking that produces anti-nutrients and free radicals which can damage cell membranes. Burnt, fried and even heavily charcoal-grilled foods can have a similar effect. These cooking methods should be limited. When frying, add a small quantity of water to cold-pressed olive oil and never allow the oil to get so hot that it smokes.

Alcohol

Alcohol has some beneficial and some detrimental effects for women with PCOS. There is now a well-documented beneficial effect from one or two units of red wine on the risk of cardiovascular disease. Like exercise, red wine increases the levels of the good (HDL) cholesterol in the blood.

The down-sides are that alcohol exerts an oestrogen-like action and can be thought of as adding to the body's oestrogen load. Also, alcohol contains a lot of refined carbohydrates which are definitely of no benefit at all.

We would suggest that while you are trying to bring symptoms under control and make big improvements, a period of abstention is very helpful. Once you are at your ideal body weight and body fat percentage and have become fitter, drinking socially in moderation is probably not only enjoyable for most women but may offer additional cardiovascular protection. Research shows that red wine contains bioflavonoids, which, together with the alcohol, is cardio-protective. Those women who have a low level of HDL cholesterol (the 'good' cholesterol) may want to take 1 to 2 units a day to raise it. But it should be remembered that exercise will also achieve this beneficial effect, and should be your first port of call as a result of the negative effects alcohol can have.

How Much Protein?

There are two important reasons for eating good quality protein. All the structures made out of protein within your body (with a few notable exceptions such as the lens of the eye) are completely remade at least once a year. Some structures are turned over even faster than this. To make new proteins you need to take in a good source.

Secondly, we now know that protein intake can modulate insulin production. Research has demonstrated that the absorption of carbohydrates and the accompanying rise in the level of blood insulin can be minimized if the carbohydrates are eaten together with some protein.

A commonly quoted figure is two portions of carbohydrate to every one portion of protein. This could potentially result in a large amount of animal protein intake, however, and this may not be so helpful because of the increased saturated fat that would also be consumed.

It is possible to eat greater amounts of vegetarian sources of protein, though when one looks at the diets of many vegetarians and measures their protein intake it is commonly very small. Without a reasonable protein intake it is not possible to increase your muscle mass. As we have seen, your muscle mass will affect your resting metabolic rate. This in turn affects the ease with which you can reduce your body fat, control your body weight and affect your symptoms.

Good sources of protein that are low in the bad (LDL) fats include chicken and turkey breast, oily fish and egg whites.

The best vegetable sources of protein are soybeans, split peas, kidney beans, peas, wheatgerm, lima beans, black-eyed peas, lentils and black beans.

How much protein you need will depend on how much exercise you do. The recommended daily allowance (RDA) of protein for sedentary individuals is 0.75 g per kilogram of body weight. However, for those who are trying to get fit and develop their muscles there is now a lot of evidence to suggest that this RDA is insufficient. The figure should be between 1.3 – 1.5 g/kg of body weight, which is twice the RDA. Everyone's individual requirement will vary.

Your protein intake should be split throughout the day, so that at every meal you take in some protein with carbohydrates from wholegrains, vegetables and fruit. This will help reduce your insulin production from the given amount of carbohydrate eaten.

Timing Your Meals

The typical way that many of us find ourselves eating is a small (or non-existent) breakfast, followed by a light lunch and then an evening meal which is the biggest meal of the day. We not uncommonly hear of people not eating anything until their evening meal, and this might not be until 8.30 in the evening. Stacking your calories like this has a number of effects. First, you are telling your body that once you have got up in the morning you are fasting. In the fasted state your body will do its best to hold on to every last calorie, as it is not too sure where or when it will get the next one. Your body achieves this very effectively by reducing your metabolic rate. Not only this, but in the fasted state, because of your brain's almost absolute requirement for glucose, you begin to break down your own muscle to provide the carbon structure to make the glucose. You cannot, unfortunately, convert fat into glucose. The net effect is a loss in muscle mass and a reduction in your metabolic rate.

Then, when you do eat in the evening, your body is now set up to store as much fat as possible away. After eating you then go to bed, so your body has little time to use any of the calories that you have just consumed.

If you were to spread your calories unevenly throughout the day in this way, which we do *not* recommend, you should at least take most of them in the morning for breakfast, or at lunch. This would avoid being in 'fast mode' during the day, and allow some of the calories to be burned off during the day's activities.

Better than this is to give your body food more regularly throughout the day, every two or three hours. Again, if we look back in history at most societies, this is naturally what humans have done.

Start the day with breakfast, have a mid-morning snack, followed by lunch, afternoon tea, then supper. All we need to get right now is what to eat at each of the meal times. Obviously they do not need to be large meals, but should combine some complex carbohydrates with a small amount of protein.

Preparation

Starting to make these changes to the way that you eat will require some preparation. Breakfast is a good meal to begin with. It is often the meal that is completely ignored. You may not feel like eating two minutes after you jump out of bed, so try and give yourself a little time to wake up before eating. Preparing something for later in the day such as a few snacks to take to work will start your digestive system working. Then eat some breakfast.

Often at work there will not be the facility to buy good quality food. Cooking a little extra the night before so you can take a few small snacks in to work with you can be very helpful. An extra (organic if possible) chicken breast, piece of salmon or pot of reduced-fat hummus together with some vegetable sticks such as carrots, celery and cucumber is simple and will work wonders at 11 a.m. or 3 p.m. as you begin to wilt,

as would some fresh or dried fruit and a handful of nuts or seeds such as
sunflower, walnuts or almonds.

For other ideas on healthy snacks see the 'Food Cravings' section in the
A–Z of Symptoms chapter.

Nutritional Supplementation

There are increasing concerns that our modern diet, high in refined
carbohydrates, sugar and non-food anti-nutrients, may no longer be (and
probably never was) sufficient to meet all our nutritional needs. Does this
mean that we should all take additional vitamins and minerals? And if
so, which ones and how much?

A nutritional supplement should be just that – a supplement to your
food, not a replacement. We are designed to obtain our nutrients from
the food we eat. In this organic form all our nutrients are well designed,
packaged, absorbed and assimilated into our bodies.

Of the man-made vitamin/mineral preparations on the market there is
vast variation. Some are good, some bad. Many preparations not only are
so poorly absorbed as to be useless, but they can also cause severe side-
effects. So, just as a drug should be considered potentially dangerous, do
not believe anyone who tells you that because a product is 'natural and
not a man-made drug it is safe'. Almost anything you can think of can kill
you, even water and oxygen.

A good example of a poor supplement, which is used by many doctors
is the iron preparation prescribed to treat anaemia. Inorganic ferrous
sulphate is often the preparation of choice. It is extremely badly absorbed
and causes quite commonly such severe gastrointestinal side-effects that
those prescribed refuse to take it in spite of debilitating anaemia.

How can you be sure that you are receiving sufficient nutrients from your
food? Without seeing a qualified medical nutritionist it is clearly difficult
to know. As we described, a poor intake of chromium, for example, may

have a detrimental effect on your insulin metabolism. So should all women with PCOS then take additional chromium?

The answer must be no. For some there may be benefit, but as with everything, more does not always mean better. And the amount required to avoid a deficiency probably does not equal the intake require for optimal function. Where does this leave us?

First, you must improve the quality of your diet to ensure it is as nutrient-rich as possible. While you are doing that, it is probably reasonable to take a good multi-vitamin and mineral preparation to support yourself while you are changing the foods that you choose to eat. This will ensure you are receiving a base-line combination of all the essential vitamins and minerals.

As our diets are typically very low in the good essential fats, the omega-3 series obtained from eating oily fish, again while you are changing your diet it would be reasonable to take 1,000 mg of EPA. Make sure it is from a reputable source, as poor quality fish oils are contaminated with heavy metals like mercury and may end up doing you more harm than good.

The only additional support you might consider would be some extra vitamin C. There is an overwhelming body of evidence to suggest that our diets provide a sub-optimal amount of vitamin C, and that a 500 mg supplementation maybe of considerable benefit, especially for those with high cholesterol or who are at risk of cardiovascular disease.

It would not be sensible to describe the use of other specific nutritional preparations, because everyone is unique and what might be found to be lacking or of benefit for one person may well not be the same for another.

Self-experimentation with high doses of nutrients can be dangerous. Nutrients and can have pharmacological actions alongside their physiological ones. For a more in-depth review of the nutritional quality of your diet and specific deficiencies you need to be individually assessed by a nutritionist, preferably one who works in a team that includes a doctor.

The aim of the nutritional principles outlined in this book is to ensure that you can make safe and sensible changes in your diet that will improve your symptoms and well-being. They are not intended to replace the individually tailored advice of a qualified nutritionist.

EXERCISE

We have discussed at some length the benefits of exercise, particularly for women with PCO/S. So how much do you do and when?

Fat-burning exercise is relatively low-intensity stuff and many people find it boring. Jogging, cycling, swimming and brisk walking have all been shown to work well as fat-burning exercises. What is not so well known is that this exercise is best done in a fasting state – that is, first thing in the morning before eating any calories. What is more, 20 minutes of low-intensity aerobic exercise performed at this time is worth 1 hour of the same exercise done at any other time of day. The reason for this is that the low levels of insulin seen first thing in the morning allow your body to access your body fat for energy to be burned by your muscles. After eating anything, even some breakfast cereals, your insulin levels will rise. Since insulin is the hormone of storage, and rises after consuming carbohydrates, it inhibits the Lyase enzymes that allow fat to be mobilized and used for energy.

So for those of you who want to burn off a few calories, try doing this straight after waking. Start off with just 5 or 10 minutes three to five mornings each week, gradually building up the time until you can complete 20 – 30 minutes in one session. An exercise bike can be very useful especially if jogging early in the morning might not be safe or it's too early to get to a gym or sports centre. You could also try finding an exercise video you are comfortable with and just doing the short warm-up routine, which usually involves some aerobic marching on the spot and a few stretches. You may well be surprised how easy it is to eat after a little exercise and a shower, even if normally you might not fancy eating so early in the day.

Some women with PCOS find that they feel terrible first thing in the morning and that exercise at this time would be very difficult. For these women it is best to start doing some exercise at a later point in the day, to allow your body to adjust. Later on, once you are feeling better, this can be moved to the earlier slot to increase the effect. Remember, starting to do something is the key.

Lastly, if you have any other concurrent medical problem please ensure that you obtain a medical opinion before embarking on a new exercise program.

Even those women who are not overweight will benefit from an exercise program. It improves your insulin sensitivity and will reduce your stress levels. Women with PCO/S have a genetic predisposition that responds well to exercise, like it or not. If you want to start simply, try getting off the bus a stop early, or cycling or walking to the supermarket instead of using the car. You could also start getting out of the elevator a couple of flights early and using the stairs the rest of the way – the same goes for the underground, subway or at train stations – choose the stairs.

Whatever you do it is important to be very careful and take it easy. Injuries are the thing that will most hold back anyone who is trying to get fit. As you get older injuries will take longer to recover from, so avoiding them is always better than having to treat them.

Once you have begun to improve your cardiovascular fitness it is then important to start a more comprehensive exercise program. You could join a gym where you can receive instruction about how to use the equipment to avoid injuries and have an individual program worked out for you. For those of you who need continual motivation, a personal trainer can be very helpful; most gyms are now equipped to offer this sort of service. Your goals will probably need to include increasing your lean body mass while reducing your percentage of body fat.

If going to a gym sounds expensive or daunting there are plenty of other good forms of exercise you can take. How about joining an aerobics, yoga or dance class such as tap dancing, salsa or even belly dancing? That way you can take a friend along for support and motivation. Or using an aerobics video at home can be useful if you enjoy it. You could also try taking up a sport you used to enjoy at school, such as tennis, basketball or badminton, so the element of competition and company takes your mind off the fact that you are doing exercise. Or try swimming – many clubs and sports centres have women-only swimming sessions where you can meet friends and chat as you swim lengths. If you enjoy swimming but feel self-conscious, you can always ask about which times of the day the pool is most quiet and try to go then. If you enjoy being outdoors, how about joining a cycling club, a walking association for a brisk country walk at the weekends, or taking up rollerblading in the park? You can also do these things on your own, of course, or with a friend.

Once you begin a regular exercise routine, you may want to reduce your morning cardiovascular workout to two or three mornings each week.

STRESS MANAGEMENT

It is impossible for most of us to avoid stress altogether – and that probably would not be healthy either – but having the ability to manage the stress in your life is a crucial part of improving the quality of your life. It is quite clear that additional stress that is poorly controlled is associated with a reduction in the quality of life and an increase in the incidence of many symptoms. Most women with PCOS have found that as the stress in their lives increases or their ability to control their stress decreases, their symptoms get worse. We have seen how the elevated levels of the stress hormone cortisol released by the adrenal gland are associated with many of the symptoms seen in women with PCOS, and also increase their degree of insulin resistance.

There are many methods that can be employed to manage the stress in your life. Exercise is particularly helpful for combating stress. Meditation, aromatherapy, acupuncture and homeopathy have all been found to be useful. It is important to find something that suits you, then use it.

Here are simple steps you can take for yourself within your day-to-day life to help lower your levels of emotional stress.

Stretch It Out

Tension can get stored in your muscles. Release those knots with a few stretches at your desk, as if you were warming up for exercise. If you feel like an idiot, lock yourself in the toilet to do it.

Breathe

If you find yourself winding up into a panic, take 5 minutes to close your eyes and take deep breaths. Once you're breathing deeply, reverse the action. Instead of breathing in as the first part of the breath cycle, push your breath out to empty your lungs and let the in-breath take care of itself. It's amazing how much deeper your breathing gets, and how calm you'll feel.

Think Positive

Writing a positive message to yourself – such as 'I have the skills to do my job really well' or 'Treat every day as a gift' – and sticking it somewhere you will see it throughout the day can actually help to keep you feeling positive.

Have a Chat

It's simple but it works. A good talk with friends helps you to let off steam. Just make sure you return the favour and do the listening when they have a problem.

Return to Sender

Write a letter to the world, getting all your gripes off your chest. Then burn it, imagining that you are getting rid of all your troubles as the smoke floats away.

Colour Up

If you feel gloomy, try putting something orange on your desk or anywhere you will see it often, as it is the colour of joy. Green is the colour of calm and serenity, so help yourself unwind by looking at a postcard of a woodland in spring.

Sleep on It
Give yourself a good night's sleep and you'll be stunned at the drop in your stress levels next day. If you find it hard to unwind, have a warm (not hot) bath before bed, or put a couple of drops of lavender essential oil on your pillow to help promote a deep sleep.

Have a Good Cry
'It's very important that people cry when they feel like it, as it's an adaptive response to stress,' says Dr William Frey, research director of The Health Partners Tear Research Centre in Minnesota. 'People feel better after crying because they're getting rid of chemicals in their tears that build up during stress.'

Under Pressure
Beat anxiety with this acupressure tip. With your hand palm up, use the fingers of your other hand to press a point on the little finger side of your arm, an inch below the wrist. Massage in tiny circles for up to 3 minutes.

Smell Yourself Well
Use the calming anti-anxiety properties of the following aromatherapy oils: lavender, clary sage, neroli, jasmine and vetivert. Dab a few drops of any one of these oils onto a tissue and inhale, or unwind in a bath with 2 to 5 drops of your chosen oil.

Flower Power
The best known Bach Flower Remedy is Rescue Remedy – take 4 drops under the tongue for any stressful emergency situation, loss of control, panic or nervousness.

Herbal Tea
Try drinking a cup of camomile or lemon balm tea, as both these herbs are famous for their soothing and revitalizing properties. You can buy them at any good supermarket or healthfood store.

Pamper Yourself

Have a massage! Find out what's on offer locally, or get a 'how to' book out from the library and persuade your partner to get the hang of do-it-yourself massages.

Massage leaves you more alert and raises concentration levels and mental agility because it boosts circulation. Give your shoulders and neck a squeeze at your desk, or organize an on-site massage company to take you and your colleagues in hand.

Try just rubbing your head and stroking your hair, or getting someone else to do it for you. It will help you to unwind. Or find an Indian head massage practitioner.

Laugh It Off

Laughter really can be the best medicine for stress – it sends feelgood chemicals whizzing around your brain to relax you. Get out your favourite funny video once a month, or make a date to visit a comedy club with a few friends.

Creature Comforts

Stroke a friendly cat or dog, or watch a goldfish swimming around its bowl and you'll probably lower your blood pressure and feel more relaxed.

Get Some Perspective

Dr Stephen Palmer, Director of the Centre for Stress Management in London, advises asking yourself what is the worst that will happen if you don't get something done, or if this situation continues. Ask yourself how important this incident will be three months from now. Ask yourself if you are making a mountain out of a molehill. 'Once you put your situation into perspective, you will feel less tense and stressed about it,' he says.

Gifts of Time

'Traffic jams and long lines at the bank or supermarket can be very frustrating – often because you feel you are wasting time that could be spent more productively doing something else,' says Dr Stephen Rechstaffen, author of *Timeshifting*. Stress will melt away if you shift your response and see the wait as 'found' time, a gift of a few moments to yourself in which to gather your thoughts and relax. Read a book, call a friend for a chat, let yourself daydream and you will feel refreshed.

Get a Move On!

Physical activity is one of the best stress-beaters around, but fitting it in to a busy day can seem destined to up your stress levels. So build exercise in – a brisk 10-minute walk at lunchtime loosens muscle tension and boosts endorphin levels to lift your mood.

Zone Out

Daydreaming is what hypnotherapist Paul McKenna calls a natural stressbusting break. Allow your mind to wander for 5 minutes if you feel truly tense. Maybe use a favourite picture or holiday postcard that you keep in the kitchen at home or on your desk at work to help you drift off.

There are more stress-busting tips mentioned in the next chapter.

Emotional Help

The emotional consequences of PCOS are often just as difficult to deal with as the physical ones. Acknowledging the emotional problems that you experience in whatever area of your life can be painful. But simply bringing them to the surface can make them seem less traumatic and easier to cope with.

In the end, your journey of coming to terms with the physical and emotional aspects of having PCOS is designed to stop you feeling like a PCOS sufferer and to get you feeling like a woman who just happens to have PCOS.

BODY IMAGE

You would have to look very hard to find someone who isn't worried about the way they look. And although many more men are beginning to come under pressure from media images and women's expectations of them, most images of naked or semi-clothed bodies displayed in public are still of female bodies.

PCOS can focus your attention even more firmly on your body than it would be even if you didn't have the condition. Putting on weight, dealing with acne, finding darkening or excess body hair, losing hair from your head, worrying about fertility or coping with infertility can all strike at the heart of your sense of womanhood and femininity.

❊ *I feel betrayed by my body. I have always wanted children and seen my body as the perfectly designed machine to provide them, but it has failed me. I feel like a failure.* Katrina, 35

❊ *I am horrified by the acne I get. I feel as self-conscious as a teenager about going out in public without lots of make-up on. And they come over my back and chest as well, so I can't wear what I want to wear because I have to cover up.* Kerri, 26

I feel manly. I'm ashamed of my moustache, and having a hairy belly button is just gross. Emily, 21

If someone looks at me, I think they are staring because I am so freakish. I used to be a size 10 and now I'm a size 18 and I feel too fat. I feel like I can't eat in public because people will look at me and think I don't deserve to be eating because I am so fat. Henrietta, 34

I don't feel like I'm a proper woman because I don't have many periods. I feel like my body isn't a woman's body because it doesn't seem to work properly. Joan, 36

I used to love my long hair. But I had to have it all cut off because it was all coming out. I looked in the mirror one day and realized my hair was straggly and thin and looked awful. But I can't help feeling I have lost my crowning glory. I don't feel as attractive any more. Rachel, 25

The depths of these women's disappointment and self-consciousness might seem extreme. But the issues they raise are very real. When your body doesn't do what you expect it to do, doesn't look as you would wish it to look and can be seen to have betrayed you in some way by cheating you out of the simple pleasure of not having to think about it (never mind being happy with it) your self-confidence takes a knock.

Most of us don't like some part of our bodies, from a nose we perceive to be crooked to a bottom we're convinced is half the size of a bus. Other people probably don't think the same thing, and see you far less critically than you see yourself. This is the difference between your body and your body image.

Restoring and maintaining a positive body image when you have PCOS can be hard, especially if you have mood swings, feel depressed or are going through trying for a baby or even starting up a new relationship. It can also be difficult if you have previously been happy with your body and you look back upon a 'golden age' when your life seemed to be just right because you were slimmer or less hairy or whatever it is you have decided was the best thing about your body at that time. This can be especially true if you have had an eating disorder in the past (eating disorders can be a trigger for PCOS, as we have seen). Body image problems can also lead women to develop eating disorders, or an unhealthy relationship with food because they are unhappy about the way they look and go about trying to change this in the wrong way (for self-help for eating disorders see the A–Z of Symptoms chapter; for further information and support groups see the Useful Addresses chapter).

There are two mental steps which are empowering and important for women wanting to help themselves feel less negative about their bodies. Letting go of your rosy image of the perfect past or the perfect future to be, and learning to be happy with how you are now is one of them. Forgiving your body for 'betraying' you is the other.

These are very difficult processes to try and work through. Counselling can help, but carrying out easier, smaller steps towards a more positive outlook can also slowly help you to feel happier about yourself.

SIMPLE STEPS TO BETTER BODY IMAGE

❋ Prune your wardrobe. Give some of your clothes to charity. If they're too small and you're keeping them there for when you lose weight, they're only making you feel guilty. If they're unflattering but you keep them because of sentimental value, take them out of your wardrobe and store them away. If they're comfy but you always feel a bit unsure about your appearance in them, put them aside for weekends around the house, or bite the bullet and get rid of them – you'll always be able to find comfy clothes that make you feel good.

❋ Stand tall. Think about your posture. You will feel more confident and look more streamlined if you stand, walk and sit properly. Try reminding yourself to sit properly at your desk on the hour every hour – you'll be surprised how quickly you develop better habits. Or take a course in The Alexander Technique to help realign your posture permanently.

❋ Exercise! Getting out for a brisk 20-minute walk (try and make sure you're slightly out of breath as you go) will make you feel instantly fitter. The buzz you get from having spent time on yourself, and achieved something you keep meaning to do, will make you feel good.

❋ Change your image. It could be a new haircut you've been dying to try, a new shade of lipstick, or thinking about mixing and matching your existing wardrobe in new combinations. Taking even half an hour to think about the way you'd really like to look will help you face the world with confidence.

❋ Talk about it. Why do you feel so uncomfortable with your body? Can you pin down particular instances that make you feel self-conscious? Do you know you focus all the unhappiness in your life on the way you look, telling yourself life would be perfect if you could only lose weight? Perhaps you could consider counselling to talk out your problems.

❋ Get treatment for PCOS. If you're not already getting treatment, go and ask for help from your doctor. Even this step will help you to feel better. If you're having treatment and it's not working or you're not happy with it, don't just carry on without asking questions – your treatment may be something your healthcare practitioner can adjust to suit you better.

SELF-ESTEEM

Body image and self-esteem are intimately linked. The danger lies in allowing your negative attitudes towards your body to colour your sense of yourself as a failure in all areas of your life. 'Low self-esteem can build gradually,' says psychotherapist Gael Lindenfield. 'You start to develop habits of not looking after yourself, choosing relationships that are not healthy, and selling out on your values.'

❄ *I know that when I first started getting acne and my periods were irregular I felt my body wasn't like a normal woman's body and I wouldn't let my boyfriends come near me, which caused the end of several relationships.* Susan, 44

Accepting that you have self-esteem problems and tackling them now can help to stop a downward spiral – deciding that you're not good enough before you start something, which means you don't make much effort with it and end up fulfilling your idea that you're not very good at it.

Although it's been said a hundred times before, accentuating the positive aspects of your life and relationships is one of the best ways to maintain self-esteem while you work through the issues surrounding your body image.

The better your levels of self-esteem in general, the better your body image will be. A strong sense of self-worth can make life feel good and full of possibilities. It's well worth putting in some effort to give you a lift.

Here are a few ideas to get you started.

❋ Acknowledge your strengths. Write out a list of all the things you know you're good at, from dealing with people on the phone at work, to making a great vegetable lasagne, or even picking up bargains. You'll be surprised at the lift it will give you to spend a few thoughts on your positive traits.

❋ Make a list. Spend a week noting down every time you feel full of self-confidence and why, and the times when you feel low on self- confidence. It could be anything from making an effort to go on a date with your partner to spend some quality time together, to agreeing to do someone a favour when you haven't got time. At the end of the week, take a look at your balance sheet and think about what you can do to boost the good times and turn the bad times around.

❋ Mirror work. 'Look in the mirror and say "I love you, I really, really love you," every day at least once,' says Louise Hay. 'It might seem very weird at first but it's all about accepting yourself as naturally lovable and giving yourself love now, rather than waiting until you lose the weight, get a new job, tell your partner what's been bugging you.'

❋ Homoeopathic remedies can help you to level out the downward spiral and decide to take positive steps.

    If a crisis leaves you weepy one minute and cheerful the next, try the homoeopathic remedy Ignatia. For someone who looks to be coping well on the surface, but underneath is full of anger andresentment, try Staphysagria. If you find yourself taking things too seriously, with anxiety, insomnia and irritability towards others, try Arsenicum album. These remedies are available in pharmacies and healthfood stores. Take them twice a day, dissolving them on your tongue. Don't take for more than 2–3 days without consulting a practitioner.

❋ The Bach Flower Remedies aim to treat a whole spectrum of emotional states. Larch is good if you are lacking in self-confidence and always believe you'll fail so don't even try. If you're convinced that you're not as attractive as other people, try Crab-apple. If you tend to take the blame for things even when they're not your fault, try Pine.

❋ Do something. If you've been promising yourself you'll start a new class at nightschool, exercise more, eat more healthily, even get a new haircut, stop putting it off and get on with it. Even if you've been meaning to clean out the fridge, or call a friend you haven't spoken to in a while, or even take the bottles taking over your kitchen to the bottle bank, get rid of the guilt by getting started. Getting through that mental block will give you a rush of good feeling and help you to start making bigger changes in your life.

❋ Step lightly. Bring fun and humour back into your life and you are guaranteed to feel better. Children laugh all the time, but as we grow into adults we grow out of the habit. It's all too easy to feel downtrodden and get stuck in a rut of complaining and focusing on the serious and downsides of life. Plan in some play time, whether it's walking the dog, watching a comedy video, phoning a friend who always makes you laugh, even sharing your in-jokes from work with your partner at home, or reading a favourite book.

❋ Congratulate yourself when you do something well. If your friend, partner or child did something they were proud of you'd congratulate them. So be kind to yourself once in a while. Tell someone you feel good about what you've achieved. Or reward yourself with something simple such as a bunch of flowers, a walk in the park or cooking your favourite meal.

❋ Learn a new language. If you think and talk about yourself in words and phrases that carry a negative message, you will sooner or later end up believing them. A powerful esteem-booster is to make a conscious effort – whenever you think of it – to clean up your language and fill it with positive, liberating messages about yourself. For instance, avoid phrases like 'I can't' or 'I'm hopeless'. Replace with something like, 'I'll do my best' or 'I'm getting better at ...' Turn 'problems' into 'challenges' and 'nervousness' into 'excitement'. Avoid 'oughts' and 'shoulds', and phrases about 'fault' and 'blame'. When something goes wrong, remember it is just one event – don't use it as a chance for a long-term self-term condemnation such as 'I always get that wrong.'

Partnerships

Feeling unattractive and having low self-esteem, as well as PCOS symptoms including emotional turmoil such as mood swings and depression, can all affect your relationships. Many women with PCOS talk about feelings of guilt when they put on weight or because their bodies have changed, and they feel they are not the person their partner was first attracted to, or are afraid that their partner finds them less desirable than before.

Some women have talked about the huge burden of feeling they have let their partner down if they have difficulty conceiving or end up not having children.

❋ *Sometimes I feel like I should tell my husband that it's OK for him to leave, that I understand that he wants children and it doesn't look like I'll be able to make his dream come true. I don't want him to leave, of course I don't, but sometimes I feel I don't have the right to expect him to stay.* Debbie, 33

Another common area of difficulty is the sense that being in a partnership should mean no secrets, and yet not wanting to tell your partner that you have to shave or wax or bleach your top lip every day; or that you take antibiotics for your acne.

❋ *In the same way that a lot of my friends would always lock the door if they were on the toilet, I always lock the door when I'm bleaching. I know he probably knows but it helps me to feel more feminine.* Angela, 35

On the other hand, some women feel that sharing their whole PCOS journey with their partner is the best thing they could have done.

❋ *I think it's really sad if people feel they can't share their intimate lives with their partners. I am still Annabel inside whether I'm upset about putting on weight or I have to shave my stomach. Dealing with what life throws at you as a couple can help you to get through it all feeling much better about yourself.* Annabel, 29

No one can really tell you what to do to get the best out of your relationship when you have PCOS. But thinking about the underlying causes of problems and insecurities can help you to isolate a problem such as a bad body image or a lack of energy, and try to focus on improving one thing at a time. And talking about your relationship and your emotional life together can help you to work out how your partner feels about your PCOS and how it affects you, your partner and your time together. You might have convinced yourself that your partner feels cheated, or has stopped fancying you because you've put on weight, only to discover that they feel you are pushing them away and they don't know what to do about it.

❀ *When Natalie found out she had PCOS she was pleased to know all the mood swings and weight had a name and it wasn't her fault, but she retreated into herself. It was like there was this thing she had to fight on her own, and I felt lost because I didn't really understand about women's health very much, but whenever I asked her she didn't want to talk about it.* Ian, 28

In the end Ian went to his doctor and asked for an information leaflet and told Natalie he'd tried to find out because he wanted them to go through it together. They are still a couple and are now trying for a baby.

It can be tempting to put a heart-to-heart on hold because you're afraid that your partner will start saying things you don't want to hear, or you'll start realizing that PCOS has nothing to do with your problems as a couple but that you're just the wrong couple and then you'll be left to deal with it on your own. But being brave and initiating discussions about your life together, or even wordlessly trying to get back into a rhythm of intimacy with your partner, can help you to discover whether you are really happy, whether you have the right support in your relationship, and whether or not PCOS has to affect your time together.

YOUR LONG-TERM SEX LIFE

Boosting Sexual Confidence

If you have a satisfying sex life as a single person, or your partnership is going as well as you expect or want it to, then stop reading this and go out and enjoy yourself.

But if you feel you want to find someone new, or your relationship has dwindled a bit, or you're not as close as you once were and you feel stuck in a rut, read on for a few ideas about helping you get back on track.

First of all you have to look at PCOS in the context of our busy modern lifestyles. It can be easy to hide behind your tiredness, symptoms and fluctuating self-esteem and use them as the reason for the sex in the relationship fizzling out, or for hiding at home and not meeting anyone new, without actually trying to work out what's going on at a deeper level. Your sex life could be affected simply by your busy life, taking care of the kids, stress at work and a hundred other things aside from PCOS.

If you feel that tackling basic day-to-day problems like never going out because you haven't got a reliable babysitter, spending lots of time sitting in front of the TV together rather than talking, worrying about money problems, or being miserable because you're in a job you hate, then sorting out these problems first could lend you or your existing relationship a new lease of life.

Back to Basics

If you are in a partnership and your life together is great apart from when you are actually together, then you probably need to do a bit more digging. Although there is a huge amount of pressure on all of us to feel that if we're not 'beautiful' our partners will be turned off by us, underneath we all know there is whole lot more to a relationship. There are core rules to attraction which involve personality, engaging conversation, fun and shared passions – and you can engage in these things whether you feel you look great or not. It is a chicken-and-egg situation – some of you may feel you really don't want to get into this sort of stuff until you feel good about your appearance. But on the other hand, getting back in touch with all these shared intimacies and injecting some variety back into your relationship can actually have the effect of helping you feel more attractive.

Here are a few ideas to get you started on building intimacy back into your relationship:

❋ Talk to each other.

It's all too easy to talk about the practicalities of everyday life without touching on how you and your partner are feeling about life, work and each other. Try making a pact for a week that as soon as you see each other at the end of a busy day, no matter how late it is, you will spend 10 minutes together to talk about the kind of day each of you had, and then another 10 minutes expressing how the day affected you emotionally. This way you can give each other support and build up intimacy, which can otherwise get lost.

❋ Get in touch.

When you have PCOS it can be difficult to engage in a sexual relationship because you're tired, you feel moody, anxious or you don't feel comfortable with your body. But a fear of intimacy can often stop you even holding hands with your partner and can shut them out. Make a conscious effort to show physical affection, and to receive it. You will be surprised at how supported and accepted this can make you feel.

❋ Enrich your partnership.

Spend some 'quality time' together, whether it's a daily chat over a cup of tea, a picnic one weekend afternoon, a walk in the park or being mischievous and spending a 'sick day' off work together.

❋ Have fun.

Sex can become a battleground for so many conflicting emotions that it's easy to forget that it – and your relationship – are

---

meant to be fun. Rekindle a level of fun in your day-to-day life – share jokes from the office, or talk about what the kids said to make you laugh, and try things together that you haven't done before, whether that's bowling, reading to each other from your favourite books, sharing the story behind a favourite photograph or even going to the cinema instead of renting a video.

Let's Talk About Sex

If you feel your intimacy levels with your partner are well established but your sex life has dwindled, try and work out the dynamics in the relationship. Do either of you want the sex back? Does one of you seem to want it more than the other?

Now is the time to try and talk to your partner about what is happening in your physical relationship. It's easier to say than it is to do, because if there's one thing that we get embarrassed about talking about it's sex, especially if it hasn't been happening for a long time. So how do you start a conversation about sex?

✳ Ask for support.

Whether in the bedroom or outside you can always ask for help in raising an issue. It helps to make the issue a shared one. For example, 'There's something I feel we need to talk about, but I'm not sure how to deal with it. Can you help?'

✳ Be forthright.

If it's easier for you to come straight to the point, that's the way to do it. For example, you could try, 'I feel like we haven't been having sex a lot lately and I'd really like us to. How do you feel about it?'

✳ Write it down.

If face-to-face talking is too nerve-wracking, try writing out your feelings and desires, because then you can say what you really feel without getting sidetracked into an argument.

> ✻ Admit you're embarrassed.
>
> For example, 'I've always found it difficult talking about sex. But our relationship means a great deal to me. I'd like us to start talking. What do you think?'

Where to Next?

Once you've started your discussion there can sometimes be a sense of pressure to start having mad passionate sex all of a sudden. This can be a fragile time, when you could both be feeling like you have to 'perform' because you've laid your sex life on the line.

With the expectation in the air it can sometimes be useful to stir up a bit of romance, whether that's going for a candlelit meal together, a walk in the rain, suggesting a bath together, or offering to massage your partner. Although it might sound corny, actually making the effort to set aside some special time together, or even just to light a few candles in the bedroom, can really help to make you feel close to your partner and start seeing them as a lover again, the one person you can share your body with.

If you feel self-conscious about things like your weight, acne or body hair, perhaps setting aside a 'date' night in advance will give you time to prepare yourself, whether that means buying a new nightie which makes you feel sexy without revealing too much, borrowing a friend's new perfume or having your tummy waxed.

It can also be helpful (and pleasurable!) to rekindle your sense of desire with masturbation. It can be easy to get into a frame of mind where you don't see yourself as a sexual being when you're not having a particularly sexy time in your relationship. But relearning the delights of your body for yourself can sometimes help you rediscover your passionate side.

Trying for a Baby

Trying for a baby can put an enormous strain on any couple, both emotionally and sexually. It changes the nature of sex from simply a source of pleasure and connection between the two of you to a physiological process with a goal in mind. This in turn brings up the concepts of success and failure, which is enough to make anyone feel nervous about sex. This tension can be increased for couples with PCOS if they are having trouble getting pregnant.

❋ *I am so desperate for a baby that I can't have sex with my husband just to enjoy it. That means you don't feel like it very much even though it's the one thing you're supposed to be doing as much as possible to try and get pregnant. My husband feels under pressure and that doesn't help – he once said feels like he's just a sperm bank, not the man I chose to spend the rest of my life with.* Jeanette, 28

Some couples who have started infertility treatment such as IVF have found that the strain on their relationship made stopping the treatment worth while.

❋ *We were so anxious and tearful and up one minute and down the next, as well as being worried by the money side of things, that after two cycles we decided to have a break to discuss whether it was worth all the heartache. Just being able to do that actually brought us closer as a couple, because we realized that however much we wanted a baby we also still wanted each other. We had a year of just being together again before we started another cycle of treatment, and it kept us going.* Carla, 37

For couples who are going through this process it is good to know that other people are, too. Joining a support group or an email chat room can be a relief.

❋ *Once I had chatted to other people about it and talked to my husband about how loads of other couples were having 'impregnation' sex, we began to actually be able to have the odd joke about it, which was a huge breakthrough. Laughing about it broke the tension and made us feel like a couple again, and helped us to have better, less mechanical sex.* Frieda, 34

You can also get information and support from organizations set up especially for people having trouble getting pregnant or coming to terms with the fact that they will not have children, and how this affects every area of life, including partnerships. To get in touch with them, see the Useful Addresses chapter.

More Help and Support for Couples

If you and your partner find it too difficult to tackle discussing the changing nature of your relationship, or how PCOS has affected it, you can go and get some support by seeing a relationship counsellor. Having a third, sympathetic person in the room can help you to start talking about things more openly, because you suddenly feel it is 'allowed'. You can also be referred to a sex therapist in particular, if that's the area of your relationship you feel you want or need to focus on.

If this seems too daunting or public, there are many useful books out there for couples wanting to sort through their problems. You could schedule an hour a week to sit and work through your problems together in the same way as you would commit to going to see a counsellor, without feeling you have to open your heart with someone else present.

The Dating Game

If you enjoy being single or you feel you just happen to be single because that's where you are in your life at the moment, then it's not an issue for you. But being a single woman with PCOS can also be hard, especially if PCOS contributed to the breakdown of a previous relationship or if it is the thing that stops you getting intimate with anyone. As well as the questions of body image and self-esteem, there are questions about how much to tell someone how soon into meeting them.

✿ *Whenever I meet someone new I don't bother telling them anything. If they like me they like me, if they don't they don't. Unless we're going to get serious I'm not going to start going on about it. It's as much for me as for him – I just want to have a good time.* Rachel, 24

✿ *I've reached a stage in my life where I'm pretty sure that every woman's body has the odd weird thing about it and so I don't care about my hairy tummy any more. If someone's really into me they won't care.* Gillian, 39

On the other hand some women feel they want to share their PCOS experience with new possible mates they meet because they feel it helps to define who they are.

✿ *I feel PCOS is the reason why I'm single now because my previous partner couldn't cope with it all. So I don't want to run the risk of getting close to someone, letting them in on my PCOS only to find that they can't cope either. The sort of person I want to be with won't be fazed by knowing.* Kelly, 31

Sadly, however, some women feel that PCOS actually stops them meeting not only new potential partners, but even new friends.

✿ *I don't enjoy being a single woman with no friends. But I just can't face the world knowing I have a stubbly chin and bad acne, and I'm not feeling particularly good about life. I feel like I'll bring people down and they won't want to go out with me again.* Alicia, 33

No one can tell you how to live your life to enjoy it the most except you. And the only way you can decide what's best is to be honest with yourself.

✿ *I realized I was getting really depressed about being single because my best friend got married. But I kind of blamed that on my PCOS, when really I feel great and I just get acne and have trouble with no periods, but in general my life isn't that different to most women I know who worry about their weight and get bad period pain and feel like they want to get married and settled down.* Annie, 29

❋ *I used to get really down about PCOS because I felt tired a lot and I didn't get regular periods so I never felt quite right in myself. But I decided it wasn't going to beat me and I refuse to let it rule my life. If people or new men ask me what's wrong, say if I cancel a date because I'm tired, then I'll tell them. But I'm me, not PCOS.* Kia, 28

STRESS-BUSTING

Coping with long-term ill health, or worries about getting ill again if you're going through a good patch, can leave you feeling stressed. If you're tired at work one day, everything seems harder; if you've got a bout of low self-esteem, the world can seem black; if you've got yet another consultation with your gynaecologist, you can end up feeling like PCOS is a never-ending problem; if your doctor won't listen your self-confidence can be shaken. There is also a lot of anger bubbling away inside women with PCOS who feel they have been treated badly by the medical profession and that life has cheated them in some way.

All the issues we have mentioned in the book, and even just the hard work of having to eat well, exercise and deal with the emotional consequences of PCOS can leave you feeling stressed, anxious, tense and tearful.

As mentioned in Chapter 10, having a good cry can help you to let go of pent-up feelings, as can talking to other women with PCOS or your partner or a good friend.

❋ *If I get a bad day when I feel PCOS is such a struggle I call up my friend Daisy who also has PCOS because there's nothing like talking to someone who knows just how you feel.* Lana, 29

❋ *My boyfriend Jim is brilliant when I get low about PCOS. At first he used to say, 'well this will make you feel better' or 'that will help' when all I wanted him to say was, 'well, gee you must feel bad sometimes,' and just let me talk. So we had a few fights about it because he said he just wanted to help, but now we have good communication and I feel better when we talk.* Chantelle, 23

Talking out your bad days is great – but learning to manage feelings of stress and tension so you don't get as many bad days is even better. It's important to start practising effective stress-busting strategies to help let go of all this emotional and physical tension, not least because high stress levels aren't good for your health.

Aside from eating well, sleeping well and being kind to yourself, here are a few practical suggestions for helping to manage stress.

❋ Relaxing therapies.

Aromatherapy, massage and meditation are all great ways to de-stress, as is reflexology. Use the Useful Addresses chapter to get in touch with your local therapist. If it's too expensive to have a monthly treatment call the training colleges near you to see if they run discount treatment packages. Or get a good book and teach yourself.

❋ Do-it-yourself aromatherapy.

Classic essential oils to combat stress include geranium, lavender, neroli and Roman chamomile. Add 3 to 4 drops to a warm (not hot) bath, or put a couple of drops on to a burner, diffuser or light bulb vaporizer to release the calming scents.

❋ Zone out.

As mentioned in Chapter 10, daydreaming is a natural stress-busting break. Allow your mind to wander for 5 minutes if you feel truly tense. Maybe use a favourite picture or holiday memory to help you drift off.

❋ Opt out.

Find places you know make you feel relaxed and spend some time there as often as you can, even if it's only 10 minutes in the park at lunchtime.

❋ Treat yourself.

Turn off the answer machine or take the phone off the hook for half an hour and just listen to your favourite music, have a snooze, watch a video or some TV, or read a book. You'll be amazed at how peaceful you can feel when you give yourself the chance to be alone.

SUPPORT NETWORKS

You can help yourself to get through bad days and celebrate good days by gathering together your own support network. This can come ready-made in the form of a self-help group or an email chat room, or it can be the web of people you talk to about your PCOS, whether penpals, your family or your buddies at work.

Even if you feel you can cope on your own, the sense of comfort you can get from knowing you have someone there to help you if you need it is very supportive.

The people in your support network need to know how you are and what PCOS is as well as how you feel about it, so that in a time of high emotion, when you're perhaps not talking clearly, they know what you mean and won't say something that makes you feel worse just because they don't know enough. So creating a useful network is as much down to you putting in some hard work, and maybe having to bring up some personal or embarrassing topics in the beginning, as it is down to the people you enlist to help you out or just listen from time to time.

When I first got ill and was just too tired and depressed to go out with my friends or spend time doing fun stuff, I almost couldn't be bothered to explain to people what was going on. But one of my friends got really mad at me and said she hated seeing me looking so ill and upset, but there was nothing she could do to reach out to me unless I told her what was wrong. So we sat down and I explained what I could and it was the best thing I could have done. I did get a bit tired of telling my story to people, partly because I felt like I was boring them as I'd heard the story so many times. But now I don't even have to mention PCOS, I can just say I'm too tired and my friends won't be upset with me. I also get stuff from magazines and newspapers from them, or friends will tell me about something they've found on the Internet. I really feel cherished by their support.' Maria, 25

The moral of this story is don't underestimate how much the people around you are happy to be there for you, or how much you may need them to be.

A–Z of Symptoms

ACNE

Having acne as an adult woman is a demoralizing experience which makes many women feel self-conscious, unattractive and low in self-esteem.

✿ *I can't wear the clothes I want to wear or be the person I really am because I am covered in horrible acne and I think if I dress attractively or make jokes that draw attention to me people will look and think, 'she's got a nerve pushing herself forward when she's got horrible skin. Who does she think will look at her?'* Karen, 33, who has battled with acne on her face, chest and back since she was a teenager

✿ *I have been married for 12 years but I am still momentarily embarrassed when my husband and I are in bed and he touches my back because of the acne and acne scars.* Helena, 37

A large percentage of women who have acne past their teens and into adulthood have polycystic ovaries. In one study, 83 per cent of the women referred to a dermatology clinic for acne were found to have PCO on an ultrasound scan, even if they didn't have any of the other symptoms associated with PCOS.

That is not to say that all women with PCOS will have acne – the figure is thought to be around 30 to 40 per cent of women with PCOS.

The cause of acne is thought to be an increase in the skin's oil production. This oil, called sebum, is made by the sebaceous glands in the skin, which react to the male hormone testosterone. Even though many women with PCOS have slightly higher levels of testosterone in their bloodstream, some women with acne seem to have no more than usual. So it seems that women with PCOS who also have acne have sebaceous glands that are extra-sensitive to the male hormone testosterone and androgens.

Once the excess oil blocks the pores it can form blackheads and attract bacteria. Pus can then collect at the site as white blood cells rush to fight off the infection.

Drug-based treatments for acne often take at least a couple of months to work, and the acne can seem worse to start with but usually gets better as long as the treatment is stuck to.

From the Pharmacy

Creams, gels and treatments applied directly on to the skin are easy to buy – check with the pharmacist to get the right one for your skin type. Most of them contain active ingredients such as salicylic acid, antibacterial benzoyl peroxide and isotretinoin, which are supposed to loosen blackheads and allow them to be shed from the skin. They also try to reduce sebum production.

From Your Doctor

For women with PCOS who have acne the usual treatment from the doctor is the contraceptive pill Dianette for at least six months. It contains a medium dose of oestrogen but also a drug called cyproterone acetate that combats the effects of testosterone in the body and helps to prevent the sebaceous glands being triggered to produce more oil.

Your doctor can also prescribe antibiotic creams or pills to reduce the number of bacteria on the skin and help calm inflammation.

If your acne definitely comes from blackheads, Isotretinoin (Retin A), a vitamin A derivative, softens and expels blackheads and can help to prevent the inflamed red spots later on.

From the Hospital

For severe acne which doesn't respond to other treatments, the drug isotretinoin (Roaccutane) can be prescribed, but only through a dermatologist. It has a dramatic effect on acne, reducing the formation of sebum and the formation of comedones, decreases the number of bacteria and thus reduces the inflammation. However, the drawbacks are the many side-effects, and the drug cannot be taken if you are or plan to be pregnant. Over time the acne may come back, but usually in a less severe form than before.

Natural Home Help for Acne

- ❀ Pure aloe vera gel is antibacterial and soothing. Some women with PCOS have reported a big improvement from dabbing the pure gel on their acne every day. It is also renowned for healing burned skin and scars, so can be put to good use on old acne sites on the skin as well.
- ❀ For angry and inflamed acne, witch hazel is cooling and soothing. Dab it directly on the acne.
- ❀ Tea tree oil is an amazing topical antibiotic, whether used neat or in creams, oils and gels. Studies have shown it is as strong as many chemical antibiotics and peroxides but it doesn't burn the skin. Pure tea tree oil is available in healthfood stores and pharmacies.
- ❀ Echinacea is one of nature's powerful antibiotics, most commonly known as a cold and flu remedy. Dab a tincture or cream on to the affected skin. From healthfood stores and pharmacies.
- ❀ Garlic is a powerful antibiotic. Grate it into your food, or take a one-a-day supplement which will also help to protect your heart health.

❀ Ketsugo is made from Isolutrol, a substance originally derived from shark's bile, but now synthesized. 'It appears to attach itself to the receptors on the sebaceous glands, regulating the production of sebum, while softening the skin,' said Dr David Fenton of St John's Department of Dermatology at St Thomas's Hospital, London.

❀ Vitamin C creams. Debate rages about whether or not vitamin C in any form can actually penetrate the skin. However, some women have found these creams useful for acne.

❀ Taking vitamin E can improve skin elasticity. Dabbing vitamin E oil on acne and scars can help them to heal. Pierce a capsule of vitamin E with a pin and squeeze out the oil to apply it.

Homoeopathic Remedies

❀ Pulsatilla – for acne which is worse at puberty and when menstruation is about to begin.

❀ Kali brom – for itchy pimples on the face, chest and shoulders brought about by hormonal change.

If you're not sure about using homoeopathic remedies straight from the shelf, consult a practitioner.

Light Therapy

Shining different types of light on the acne, from UV to simply coloured light, can help. Ask your dermatologist about it.

ALOPECIA

See **Hair Loss**

BREAST PAIN

Tender, lumpy, painful or hardened breasts can be the result of hormonal imbalances and fluctuations, especially in the run up to a period.

Evening primrose oil has been shown to be so effective in tackling breast pain and tenderness that UK doctors can prescribe it for women with this problem. It is prescribed under the brand name Efamast. The dose recommended by doctors is around 1,000 mg per day.

You can also try starflower oil (also known as borage oil), linseeds (flax seeds) and blackcurrant seed oil. Vegetarians need to check that their capsules don't use gelatin, or can take the oil neat.

Gentle self-massage using evening primrose oil or borage (starflower) oil can also help.

DEPRESSION

Many women with PCOS feel low and depressed at some time. This can be to do with the hormonal cycles in the body (think of how many women get tearful and depressed with PMS) or simply with feeling overwhelmed by various problems the condition can throw up, from chronic fatigue to low self-esteem or fertility issues.

Don't forget, however, that there are also other types of depression which may have nothing to do with PCOS itself, such as reactive depression due to a life event such as bereavement or job loss; post-natal depression (PND) after the birth of a child, Seasonal Affective Disorder (SAD), which comes from a lack of natural sunlight; and biochemical depression as a result of a chemical imbalance in the body, sometimes due to a nutritional deficiency. Some people also experience depression as a result of an allergic reaction.

Here we explain some of the more talked-about modern treatments for depression. But it is always important to find out the type of depression before beginning any form of treatment, so if you feel that you are consistently at a low ebb and not just experiencing an occasional low mood you must seek professional guidance before starting any treatment. (See the Useful Addresses chapter for contact details of helpful and informative organizations.)

Perhaps the most talked about anti-depressant is Prozac. Prozac can be prescribed by your doctor if you have symptoms such as loss of self-esteem and inappropriate feelings of guilt and unworthiness, loss of interest in any activity, sleep and appetite disturbances, excessive fatigue, or difficulties with thinking straight or concentration.

Prozac takes around three to six weeks to start working, is less likely than traditional anti-depressants to cause sleepiness, low blood pressure or irregular heartbeat, and even a substantial overdose is not likely to be fatal. However reported side-effects include anxiety, headaches, stomach upsets, skin rashes, insomnia, lowered sex drive and alcohol cravings, and it can trigger manic episodes in those predisposed to bipolar disorder (manic depression).

There are many other anti-depressants which your doctor can prescribe for you, along with instructions on how much to take and for how long. Be aware that withdrawal symptoms can sometimes occur if antidepressants are stopped suddenly – this is something worth asking your doctor about when you are trying to decide whether to take antidepressants.

St John's Wort

St John's Wort (Hypericum perforatum), the herb billed as nature's Prozac, has the ability to work as an effective antidepressant – so much so that it is now prescribed by German doctors more often than antidepressant drugs. Although there is still argument over how it *actually works, many people who take it are just glad that it does. A recent overview of 23 clinical trials into St John's Wort and depression was carried out by Klaus Linde and colleagues and published in the famously rigorous British Medical Journal, declaring Hypericum extracts to be 'significantly superior' to placebo, and indeed, 'similarly effective' to standard antidepressants. Reported side-effects include mild nausea and extra skin sensitivity to sunlight, but unlike many antidepressant drugs, St John's Wort has not been found to lower sex drive or impair the ability to experience orgasm.*

There are many brands of St John's Wort on the market, which can vary in strength and potency. The dose of a total of 900 mg of this product daily has been shown by studies to be effective in counteracting mild depression. Visiting a registered medical herbalist for a tailor-made prescription is another way to make sure you are getting the correct dose.

Bear in mind that if you decide to treat your PCOS and all its symptoms herbally, St John's Wort may be simply one of many herbs prescribed by a medical herbalist in a treatment tailor made for you. To find out more about the herbal approach to depression or PCOS, see the Useful Addresses chapter for contacts.

Vitamins and Minerals

Vitamin B_6 is famous for helping to lift PMS depression, and your doctor may be happy to prescribe this for you if your low moods tend to coincide with your cycle. All the B vitamins are essential for a healthy nervous system, with deficiencies being linked (by some scientific papers) to depression. You and your healthcare practitioner (such as your doctor or a nutritional therapist) may feel it is worth taking a B vitamin-complex supplement.

A zinc deficiency has also been noted in some people with depression. This mineral is also essential for a healthy reproductive function.

Magnesium supplementation has also been hailed by many women with PMS as a good answer to their symptoms. It is also useful for helping to prevent a low mood and dizziness.

Homoeopathy

Qualified homoeopaths will work out the best treatment for you according to your individual emotional and physical make-up.

Having said this, common remedies include Aurum if the person feels totally worthless, suicidal and disgusted with themselves; Ignatia if the depression follows deep grief or a failed relationship; and Pulsatilla if the person bursts into tears at the slightest thing and wants a great deal of reassurance and attention.

Bach Flower Remedies are homoeopathic preparations made from flowers which deal specifically with emotional well-being. Anecdotal evidence suggests they can help people to come to terms with feeling low and move through a crisis to a more stable mood. Gorse can be used for a sense of hopelessness; Mustard for depression which has no identifiable cause; and Honeysuckle for people whose thoughts keep turning to happier times in the past.

Counselling

Talking confidentially about your problems can give you a chance to release any fears, phobias and anxieties safely. Counsellors are professionally trained in listening and helping to clarify problems.

Different types of counselling are offered, such as psychotherapy, person-centred counselling, psychoanalysis, etc. To find out more about each type and work out which one is for you, consult the Useful Addresses chapter.

Cognitive Behavioural Therapy (CBT) is a way of helping you to assess your thought patterns, realize where the negative thoughts are coming in your life, and working at ways to change your learned responses to certain situations so they are more positive in the future.

Self-help to Lift Your Mood

❈ Ask for support. Don't fall into the trap of thinking you have to be superwoman all the time. If you are going through PCOS with friends, family or a partner it can be rewarding for them to be able to help you in some way, whether that's lending a sympathetic ear or helping you out with the shopping. If you don't feel you want to share with people you already know, how about joining a support group or signing up to a email chat site so you know you're not alone?

❈ Have a good cry. If you feel like crying, don't always make yourself hold it in. It can be a relief to let out all the pent-up emotion, and a good cry leaves you feeling calmer and more able to deal with the situation at hand.

❈ Laughter sends happiness chemicals called endorphins whizzing around your body to make you feel naturally high. So do something to get you chortling, from watching a favourite comedy video to calling a friend who always makes you chuckle.

❈ Colours can lift your mood. Try looking at or wearing orange, which is associated with joy and energy by alternative practitioners called colour therapists.

❈ Cut down or cut out alcohol when you feel low, as it acts as a depressant.

❈ Pamper yourself with treats such as an aromatherapy massage or a bath at home, a facial at a salon or in your own bathroom, a night out with friends, a walk in the park, a day at the coast. These things can make us feel much better but we rarely give ourselves over to the enjoyment.

❈ Set some goals. Achievement, however small, is vital to helping you tackle low moods. But be realistic – start small, with things like cleaning the bath if it's been bugging you, giving yourself a proper lunch break every day if you never quite manage it, calling your mother on a Sunday. You will feel lighter at heart when you do what you have set out to do.

DIABETES

Diabetes mellitus is caused by a lack of insulin, a hormone manufactured by the pancreas. Insulin is responsible for the absorption of glucose into liver and fat cells, and the muscles, which all need it for energy. If there is too little insulin, glucose levels in the blood rise, as the cells which need the sugar have no insulin to help them absorb it.

Symptoms of diabetes include thirst, need to urinate a lot, weight loss, fatigue, hunger, weakness and apathy.

Type I diabetes, or insulin-dependent diabetes (IDDM) occurs usually between the ages of 10 and 16, in people who cannot produce insulin. Insulin must be given artificially through injections.

Type II diabetes, non-insulin-dependent diabetes (NIDDM), also known as 'late onset' or 'age onset' diabetes, usually occurs in people aged over 40, especially when they are overweight. This is the type of diabetes which women with PCOS are at an increased risk of developing. Some experts suggest the increase is as much as ninefold.

People with type II diabetes have plenty of insulin in the body but their tissues are insensitive to it and don't use it well (a problem also called insulin resistance), which results in a slow development of the same symptoms as in diabetes type I.

Why Do Women with PCOS Get It?

With PCO/S, insulin levels are raised much more steeply. And although there are higher levels of insulin in circulation, at tissue level these remain the same, a state called insulin resistance, which is linked to a higher risk of developing diabetes type II, or 'late onset' diabetes.

Dietary Prevention

Diabetes can cause nerve damage, contribute towards heart disease, arterial disease in the legs, high blood pressure, sight problems including blindness, and kidney failure – so if you have PCOS and any of the symptoms mentioned above it is worth asking your doctor to carry out blood and urine tests.

If you have diabetes, your doctor can advise you on a diet to help reach or maintain both a healthy weight (as excess weight makes diabetes worse) and steady levels of blood glucose, as well as give you drugs to combat insulin resistance if these are needed.

Your doctor can also monitor your progress with checks on weight, blood pressure, eyes, heart and feet, and can help you to deal with any complications which arise. You should tell your doctor if you are planning to try for a baby, as you may need to take on board special advice.

You can also take care of yourself by carrying out these simple steps:

❋ Get clued up by contacting support groups and information organizations (see the Useful Addresses chapter).

❋ Be strict with your diet. Don't tempt yourself to eat sweet things by buying them for other people in your household. Try new recipes so you find some healthy meals you really enjoy.

❋ Exercise. Doing 30 minutes of walking four times a week will help keep weight down and could help with glucose control.

❋ Look out for low blood sugar, which can cause fainting or even coma. Symptoms include light-headedness, anxiety, palpitations, hunger, panting and sweating.

❋ Find out about nutritional supplements. Read about them, see a qualified nutritional therapist or ask your local diabetes association and your doctor about supplementing with:

    ❋ vitamin B_1, which is used to metabolize glucose, or

    ❋ magnesium, which is needed for sensitizing your tissues to insulin

> �֍ chromium, which influences your tissues' response to insulin, or
> ✷ zinc, which is water-soluble and can be lost in the increased urine, or
> ✷ essential fatty acids (EFAs), which can help to keep the eyes healthy.
> ✷ Try autogenic training alongside your treatment, a form of mediation which can help to control blood sugar levels and blood pressure.

EATING DISORDERS

Although eating disorders are actually implicated in the development of PCOS, some women with PCOS feel they have developed abnormal eating patterns because of their condition.

✷ *I feel so depressed about my weight, my tiredness, my acne and excess hair that I binge eat. I know it's the last thing I should do because I feel really guilty and miserable afterwards, but when I feel low a chocolate bar seems like the ideal way to treat myself.* Marie, 29

✷ *I hate my body. If I so much as look at a cream cake I put on weight. So I don't eat them. And I don't eat much else, either. After being overweight in my early teens when I started my periods, and I suppose the PCOS kicked in, I found a real sense of achievement by not eating. I felt better being thinner and I felt I was getting one back on my body which had made me so miserable by growing hairs where they shouldn't be and making me fat. I am working through what has become an addiction to starving myself with my doctor at the moment. But I am scared that eating normally will make me really fat and even more hairy.* Jay, 19

Women's relationships with food are often very complicated, whether they have PCOS or not. Knowing that an increase in your body weight can make the symptoms worse when you do have PCOS can make you feel cheated, like you should be on a constant diet, starving yourself of treats. In the same way that dieters find themselves constantly thinking about food they are not allowed to eat, women with PCOS can feel drawn to eating things they are 'not allowed' to have.

The stories above, and many others like them, also show that many women with PCOS see their bodies as their enemies, the source of everything that is bad about their lives, whether that is because they have problems with weight, excess hair, acne, a lack of periods or are struggling with fertility issues. Denying your body the very thing it needs to stay alive can make you feel as if you are controlling it, and moves your sense of yourself away from your body and into your head – in other words, you become more and more detached from, and in control of, the body which you view as the enemy. This may give psychological relief so powerful that it becomes addictive and destructive.

Depression and food are also common companions. In the same way that some hot apple pie on a cold winter's day made you, as a child, feel loved and cozy, treating yourself to a chocolate bar, a slice of cake or a dessert in a restaurant can make you feel in a better mood because it makes you feel loved. Loving and treating yourself to pleasurable things when you have PCOS is very important, but doing so with food can lead to feelings of guilt and even more depression, and so the cycle starts all over again.

For some women with PCOS the need to eat carbohydrates, or having a sweet tooth, can actually be a result of the insulin metabolism being out of synch, in the same way as it is for people with diabetes. There are ways to help deal with this (see Food Cravings, below). However, if you feel your relationship with food is unhealthy primarily because of an emotional reaction to your life or your body, then finding some help is important.

Positive steps you can take
- ✽ You can share your story with other women who have been through the same thing by joining a support group, either in your local area or on the Internet.
- ✽ You can also find help and support through eating disorders organizations and specialist centres. (For contact details see the Useful Addresses chapter.)

❋ Your doctor should be able to put you in touch with a qualified dietitian if you feel this would be useful.

❋ Your doctor can also help you to find a qualified counsellor who specializes in eating problems or, if your unhealthy attitude towards food comes from an experience such as dealing with infertility, you may want to ask for a counsellor who can help you with that. If you don't want to see your doctor to ask for this help, you can do some research to find a qualified counsellor in your area. (See the Useful Addresses chapter.)

❋ Starting to have treatment for your PCOS can also be helpful if you are not already doing so. If you are already taking steps to change this but feel the right sort of progress isn't being made, talk to your healthcare practitioner about this. Perhaps your treatment can be modified in some way to help it become more effective and help your body to get back towards a more healthy balance.

EXCESS HAIR

Having excess hair on your body in places that are usually associated with men, such as the face/neck, chest, back, stomach, buttocks, arms, thighs, feet and toes is called hirsutism. A large number of women with PCOS struggle with this emotional rollercoaster of a problem, which they often find too embarrassing to go and seek help for.

❋ *I can't describe the misery of shaving every morning before my boyfriend gets up. I hate doing it, it makes me feel sick and unfeminine, but I'm too scared to go and see my doctor because I feel like a freak.* Cherie, 23

❋ *I hate having hairy legs in the summer. I am constantly worried that if I wear sandals someone will notice I have hairy or stubbly toes.* Justine, 36

In women with PCOS the hair follicles seem particularly sensitive to the male hormones called androgens, which circulate in the bloodstream. This can stimulate hair growth in areas usually associated with men.

Body hair in women is a hugely taboo subject – most women even without PCOS have some body hair. Many Asian and Mediterranean women have more body hair than northern Europeans, while Chinese and Japanese women often have less. So concepts of what is 'excess' hair and what is 'normal' are often difficult to define – what seems perfectly acceptable to one woman may seem unacceptable to someone else.

If your body hair makes you feel uncomfortable, embarrassed or miserable about your body there is plenty you can do to help sort it out. Unfortunately, it all costs money. (This is true even in the UK, because no treatment such as electrolysis is yet available on the NHS. The psychological side-effects of this symptom are not yet recognized as severe enough to warrant treatment, although there is also a move in some UK clinics, such as St Mary's in London, to have a beautician on site who can advise women in efficient ways of dealing with the hair cosmetically.) Also, horror stories about unsympathetic doctors are not uncommon. But there are also many professionals in the hair-removal industry who are very sympathetic and do their job well. They are trained to help women with body hair problems and will not be shocked or disgusted by whatever you feel embarrassed about. They are there to help, so if you haven't sought out a treatment because you are embarrassed, don't deny yourself.

Ideally, controlling hirsutism will be down to getting the hormonal balance right through healthy eating and exercise, but your doctor – and practitioners such as herbalists – can also help.

Contraceptive Pill

The contraceptive pill can be an effective way to tackle the problem of excess hair. Your doctor will discuss the right type of medication for your symptoms. As with any form of treatment, it's advisable to be monitored regularly while taking any form of drug.

A combined oral contraceptive with oestrogen and progestogen (synthetic versions of female sex hormones) can help decrease the amount of androgens in the blood and made in the ovaries. Also used are oral contraceptives containing a type of progestogen which blocks the effects of androgen hormones and reduces the amounts made by the ovaries.

Glucocorticoids are another type of drug used to lower the amounts of male hormones in the blood, stopping the adrenal gland from making androgens.

It usually takes several months before you start to see any results from taking medication.

Exercise

Exercise can improve hirsutism, because the fitter you become the lower your body fat and the better your insulin and glucose control. Less hyperinsulinaemia means less drive to the ovary to produce additional testosterone.

Herbalism

A combination of herbs can be effective in treating PCOS, so that when the hormones are back in balance the hair growth can lessen. The most common herb used specifically for excess hair in women is Saw Palmetto, although it's important to remember that it is best to be taken in combination with other herbs and prescribed by a qualified medical herbalist. Saw palmetto is used mainly to treat prostrate problems in men, but its pharmacology suggests it could be useful in the treatment of hirsutism and androgen excess in women.

Hair Removal

This is often a time-consuming and expensive business, because the hair seems to grow back very quickly and needs constant attention. If you are looking for long-term hair removal, the methods are often expensive, but it is worth considering how much you spend on razors, bleaches and depilatory creams every year in money and time, and adding that up to compare with the price of a permanent removal treatment.

Shaving, depilatory creams, bleaching, plucking/tweezing and waxing are well-known methods. You may have to experiment to find which is most comfortable/satisfactory for you.

Epilators are hand-held devices used like an electric razor, but they pluck hairs out rather than shaving them. It can be painful and the plucking action can sometimes encourage stronger hair regrowth.

Electrolysis

Needle electrolysis uses an incredibly fine needle or probe inserted into the hair follicle and a small electrical current sent down to the root so that the heat kills it. The dead loose hair is then discarded with tweezers. This form of electrolysis is called diathermy.

Galvanized electrolysis requires you to hold a metal rod to create an electrical current at the base of the follicle, which causes a chemical reaction with the water there, killing the root and loosening the hair. This method has a higher success rate than diathermy.

Electrolysis can provide very long-term and often permanent hair removal. However, it is very slow so not ideal for large areas of hair, can be painful and, most seriously, can cause scarring of the skin if not carried out by a well-trained operator. It also requires commitment – you have to go back very regularly, at least once a week, often for a minimum of six months, depending on the individual, to see effective, long-term results. Many therapists say that if you cannot afford the time to commit to this, it is not worth spending the money.

Transdermal electrolysis transmits an electrical current to the hair follicle through a special gel applied to the skin. This current creates a chemical reaction at the hair's root, changing the water and salt there to sodium hydroxide which dissolves the follicle. Dead hairs are then tweezered away. Transdermal electrolysis is quicker than traditional electrolysis, as all the follicles under the gel can be treated at the same time; hair removal is long term and often permanent; it feels like a prickling, tickling sensation rather than being painful. However, it still takes commitment and regular appointments for a long period of time – often at least six months – to make it worth the money.

Laser Hair Removal

Laser hair removal uses a powerful beam of light focused on the area to be treated for only a fraction of a second. The dark colouring in the hair (melanin) absorbs the light energy and transmits it down the hair shaft into the follicle, where it destroys the cells. It is most effective on fair skins with darker hairs. It is not suitable for black or suntanned skins.

Some people have reported burns and scarring as a result of inappropriate treatment. It's also important to note that anyone can purchase a laser, as there are no regulations governing who can buy one, so it's best to go to a clinic with a doctor or nurse experienced in using the equipment.

Epilight

Epilight also uses light energy, but is not the same as a laser because it uses visible light pulses which can be adjusted to different frequencies and so penetrate the skin to different depths, in order to treat hair follicles growing deeper down in the skin, for example along the bikini line.

However, Epilight works in the same way as a laser because the melanin in the hair absorbs the light energy and transfers it to heat which travels down the hair shaft and disables the new cells. It is said to be more gentle than a laser and can work on all skin types, including black skin, though currently women with darker skins are most likely to get treatment in the US.

It has a very high success rate for permanent hair removal after as few as four or five treatments for some hair, but can be very expensive. Most therapists can guarantee around 70 to 80 per cent permanent hair removal.

Soundwave Treatment

Epil-pro uses the power of soundwaves to destroy cells at the base of the hair follicle. Sterile tweezers transmit the sound waves down the hair shaft, and glide along the skin to treat hairs quickly. You would have to go around every two to three weeks to start with for the first six to eight sessions, and then less frequently depending on your hair type. It has a good reputation with women who have hormonally-triggered hair growth.

It costs the same as electrolysis treatments, but is generally quicker.

Hair Retardants

Hair retardants are body lotions, moisturizers or aromatherapy preparations which can be massaged into areas of skin which have been treated to remove the hairs in order to try and encourage finer or lighter regrowth. Ask at your local beauty salon or pharmacy.

FAINTING AND DIZZINESS

Getting adequate good quality sleep can help to reduce this symptom, as can taking a magnesium supplement. Lying down is the best way to help you feel better, as it stops the blood flow draining from your head.

You should ask your doctor for a test for anaemia, and also be aware of the risks of developing diabetes which are linked to PCOS, as dizziness can be a symptom of low blood sugar.

FATIGUE

Although many doctors don't yet recognize fatigue as a symptom of PCOS, many women with the condition report feeling very tired a lot of the time and needing to sleep for longer hours.

This could be linked to hormones if you consider the idea of unopposed oestrogen. As we have seen, in a menstrual cycle when ovulation does not take place (something which can happen fairly often in women with PCOS), the corpus luteum does not develop to pump out progesterone. With no progesterone and rising levels of oestrogen from the maturing egg follicles, there is a lot of oestrogen circulating, which can be called 'unopposed oestrogen' because no progesterone has kicked in to balance it out.

Dr Steven R Goldstein, Associate Professor of Obstetrics and Gynaecology at New York University's School of Medicine, says that research has shown that this 'unopposed' oestrogen can be responsible for physical symptoms including salt and fluid retention, low blood sugar levels, blood clotting, altered thyroid hormone function leading to weight gain and/or feelings of exhaustion, and increased production of body fat and a sluggish, 'low-energy' feeling.[1]

So, regaining a regular menstrual cycle by treating your PCOS and managing it with self-help measures such as diet and exercise could actually help to get rid of the tiredness, too.

Diabetes and insulin resistance can also play a part in creating tiredness, especially if you are slow to get going in the mornings.

Your diet has a big part to play in keeping energy levels constant and avoiding the afternoon slump. Following a healthy eating plan with plenty of fresh fruits and vegetables, wholegrains such as brown rice and wholemeal bread, and protein such as soya, pulses and lean organic meat can all help.

Fatigue can also be linked to emotional factors such as depression – when you feel low your energy is often sapped and feelings of listlessness and lethargy can take over. Wanting to stay in bed and sleep a lot is one of the signs of depression. If you think this could be something to do with your tiredness, go and see your doctor. Also see Depression, above.

Other baseline conditions to rule out with your doctor and nutritional therapist include thyroid problems, anaemia, vitamin and mineral deficiencies, food intolerances and allergies.

Tips for More Energy

✽ Getting good quality sleep is essential – for simple tips on achieving this see Sleep Problems, below.

✽ Gentle exercise can help you to feel more awake and energized. If you can go for a walk at lunchtime or more places on foot instead of by bus or car, this could help to give you a boost.

✽ If you find it hard to wake up in the mornings, try adding a couple of drops of lime essential oil to your bath, or use lemon or peppermint which can help to uplift and invigorate you.

✽ Herbal teas won't give you more energy, but a cup of peppermint or lemon and ginger can help you feel a bit more refreshed and awake.

✽ Colour therapists use orange to inspire joy and energy as well as recommending it as a good colour for women with fertility problems to wear or look at. Invest in an orange T-shirt or keep some oranges on your desk (which will also encourage healthy snacking habits).

✽ Therapies which have helped to boost energy include nutritional therapy, acupuncture, shiatsu and aromatherapy massage.

Supplementing Your Diet

If diet and lifestyle issues are causing fatigue, no supplement is going to change that. Herbs are not essential, but good nutrients are. Maybe even taking a multivitamin could help to raise your energy levels.

B vitamins are a good basic energy supplement – along with vitamin C they are involved in healthy adrenal gland function, so if you are stressed it's worth considering supplementing with a B vitamin complex, as these vitamins are often deficient in a refined Western diet. B vitamins are especially good for people who are fatigued and also have skin problems.

Adding energy tonics to your diet may also help. CoQ10 is an important nutrient within the body's energy production processes. It can be very useful if you are obese or extremely fatigued, but should be taken under the guidance of a nutritional therapist.

Ginseng is of most use for people convalescing or under major stress – these people benefit the most. Supplementing with ginseng needs to be considered on an individual basis with a qualified practitioner, as there are different types. Korean ginseng is most stimulating, so exercise caution if you have high blood pressure or oestrogen-related hormonal problems. All types will be beneficial if the lack of energy is stress-related.

FLUSHING

See **Hot Flushes/Flashes**

FOOD CRAVINGS

Many women with PCOS suffer from food cravings, particularly for sugary or carbohydrate types of food. It is not always sweet foods since carbohydrate rich foods include pasta, bread and rice. The reason for these cravings may well be due to their insulin response to eating these foods. The body needs to control the blood glucose level within a fairly small normal range. Outside this range your brain does not function very well. This is the reason why diabetics become unwell when their blood glucose is either low and they become unconscious, or too high when they become confused and disorientated. To achieve this your body looks at the rate of absorption of the glucose from the intestine and makes an appropriate amount of insulin. If there is a large amount of glucose coming in after a big meal you make a lot of insulin. If there is a small amount of glucose entering it you make a small amount of insulin.

Insulin causes the glucose that has been eaten to be stored, thereby keeping the blood level constant. It first stores the glucose in the liver and muscles as glycogen, and any excess is stored as body fat. However, as we have discussed, women with PCOS can make slightly more insulin that women without. This leads to the tendency to store calories away as body fat. The higher the level of insulin produced, the faster the glucose will be stored away and the faster the level in the body will fall. As the blood glucose level falls many of us initially feel tired and sleepy then hungry, craving something to bring back up our blood glucose again – sugar or carbohydrate cravings.

This situation can then be exacerbated by the choice of carbohydrate. Refined carbohydrates cause a more rapid rise and fall in the blood glucose leading to more body fat and worse food cravings. To reduce this tendency the choice of carbohydrate is crucial. The combination of eating some protein with each meal or snack further aids the situation by slowing down the rate of absorption of the glucose and therefore minimizing the insulin production and the rapid swings in blood glucose.

Your Questions Answered

Can chromium supplements beat food cravings?
Chromium is a mineral required for normal insulin action. It has been well documented that a great number of people may not consume an appropriate amount of chromium from their diet, and this leaves them depleted. In this depleted state their insulin may not be able to exert its usual effect.

Supplementation in insulin-resistant individuals and non-insulin-dependent diabetics has been shown to improve insulin sensitivity and reduce insulin resistance.

It is possible to have your chromium levels assessed. A good technique appears to be assessing the levels deposited in your hair, though there are also blood tests available. Hair mineral analysis is simple and non-invasive and offers assessment of all the minerals and also toxic heavy metals such as mercury, lead and cadmium, all of which have a negative effect on your health and fertility.

No one has yet performed a study to assess if chromium supplementation will reduce sugar cravings in women with PCOS. However, for women with PCOS who are insulin resistant and are chromium depleted, it is likely that improving their diet to include more of the rich sources of chromium such as brewer's yeast, wholemeal bread, rye bread, chilli, oysters, chicken, cornmeal, bananas, carrots, oranges, green beans, cabbage, mushrooms and strawberries will help their cravings. Short-term supplementation with chromium while making dietary changes can also be useful.

Does chromium work as a weight loss tool?
For those who are relatively chromium deficient it will certainly help weight loss.

Do high insulin levels increase appetite?
High insulin stimulates appetite, therefore any dietary restrictions need to be palatable, realistic and manageable. Instead of waiting for long gaps between three big meals a day, try five smaller meals to keep blood sugar regulated and reduce cravings for sweet, high-fat foods.

Can Metformin help to stop carbohydrate cravings?
Metformin can reduce appetite in some people, but it also makes some people feel nauseous, so it is difficult to tell whether it works or simply stops you eating because you feel ill. Anecdotally there are cases where women have felt better after six months on metformin, come off it and put their weight back on.

The use of Metformin as an appetite suppressant is not readily available in the UK. Until there is good evidence from controlled studies you will only get a few specialists working in the area who are prepared to prescribe it in this way. Doctors are unlikely to do this.

Practical Tips

❀ Don't go shopping when you're hungry, as you'll end up buying the snack foods you fancy eating at that moment. If your cupboard is piled high with sweet snacks, you will eat them.

❀ Stock up on healthier snacks. Ready-to-eat dried fruits such as prunes may sound unglamorous but are actually really tasty and intensely sweet. You can also try papaya chunks, pineapple, pears and peaches – but always check that there isn't added sugar listed in the ingredients.

❀ Get in some hot chocolate powder and make yourself a cup with skimmed milk or soya milk.

❀ Explore your healthfood store – rice cakes in large and snack sizes can be a tasty, crunchy snack as long as they're made from wholegrain brown rice. Add a chopped banana or a bit of pure fruit spread (check for no added sugar) and you'll be pleasantly surprised.

❀ For a comfort fix, get the hang of making a quick bowl of oatmeal porridge with skimmed milk, soya milk or water – easy in the microwave. Add raisins, nuts, fresh chopped fruit and a drizzle of honey or brown sugar.

❀ Keep fresh fruit, dried fruit and healthy snacks such as carrot sticks near your desk at work so you don't give in to the temptation to get yourself a chocolate bar when you feel the need of a quick fix.

❀ Sniffing vanilla essential oil is supposed to help prevent cravings for sweet foods such as chocolate. Choose a vanilla-based perfume or dab a couple of drops on to a tissue and inhale it when you feel the need.

HAIR LOSS

Otherwise known as alopecia, hair loss can be one of the effects of PCOS. There are different types of alopecia, some resulting in total baldness, but this is not what women with PCOS get – if they do it's not down to PCOS.

Women with PCOS get a gradual all-over thinning of the hair, where hair becomes gradually 'see through' – the sort of hair which appears as a fine fuzzy halo when a light shines on it. This is called alopecia androgenetica, and is the female version of male-pattern baldness.

❋ *Women with PCOS get hair loss and thinning due to excess androgens in the bloodstream, perhaps predisposing genetic factors and even the Pill. Mostly, women with PCOS first notice thinning hair on the top of the head, but the shedding may be variable due to when ovulation occurs and when it doesn't.* Dr David Fenton, Consultant Dermatologist at St Thomas's Hospital, London

Dr Fenton doesn't advise not taking the Pill, but says women with PCOS should be aware that stopping it, starting it and even changing brands can cause an increased shedding of hair, though this may well even out as the body adjusts to the new hormonal balance and new hair growth cycles begin.

Therefore, balancing out the hormonal cycles in PCOS is the best way to tackle the problem.

Scalp massage (easy when you're shampooing your hair) can be useful, especially if combined with essential oils. Scottish researchers recently found that 44 per cent of alopecia patients massaging their heads daily with a mix of thyme, rosemary, lavender and cedarwood oils in a carrier oil found a significant improvement in their symptoms after 7 months, compared with just 15 per cent of those using carrier oils alone.[2]

For more help contact the alopecia associations listed in the Useful Addresses chapter.

HIRSUTISM

See **Excess Hair**

HOT FLUSHES/FLASHES

This is a symptom linked to menopause and hormonal fluctuation and can be helped by magnesium supplementation, making sure you get a good diet so it is rich in vital nutrients, and helping to get your hormones back in balance with whatever treatment you are taking for your PCOS. If you are going through a patch of excessive flushing, try and wear layers of clothes when you go out so you have easy control over your temperature.

✻ Cut out the nicotine. Smokers suffer greater severity of symptoms because smoking inhibits both circulation and hormone production.
✻ Reduce your consumption of sugar, salt and junk foods – they can cause fluid retention and inhibit the uptake of nutrients in food.
✻ Avoid hot drinks, alcohol and spicy foods – all aggravate the problem.
✻ Although it seems like adding fire to fire, taking cayenne pepper in moderation can help.
✻ Vitamin E, one of the fat-soluble vitamins, has been found to be helpful in reducing hot flushes in pre- and post-menopausal women. Good sources of vitamin E include unrefined corn oil, sunflower and other seeds, peas, wheatgerm and oily fish such as sardines.

INFERTILITY

What is infertility? Simply put, infertility is when a woman cannot have a baby. But many women with PCOS are not infertile, they just have some problems getting pregnant. Doctors will usually not investigate for any problems until a couple have been trying to conceive for a year, or even two if they are younger than 30. This is because many 'normal' women and healthy couples can take at least a year to get pregnant anyway.

If 100 couples decided to try and conceive in the next year, at the end only 75, or 75 per cent, will have been successful. If the 25 couples who did not conceive went on to try for another year, at the end of the second year just less than 75 per cent of the 25 couples will have conceived. Those 7–10 remaining couples who did not conceive would then be said to have a problem with their fertility. That's about 1 in 10 couples.

The investigations that are performed (see below) are invasive and some of them uncomfortable, not to mention the time, worry and expense they involve.

For women who know they have PCOS things can be slightly different from the figures we have just given. To conceive you need to ovulate. If you are not having a regular period then it is more likely you are not ovulating – or, if you are, that you cannot predict when this will be. In a normal 28-day cycle ovulation occurs about 14 days after the first day of your period. There is some variation around this, and most doctors suggest that the fertile week would run from about day 10 to day 17 of a 28-day cycle. If your cycle is 26 days and regular, your fertile week would be from day 8 to 15; if your cycle is 32 days long, your fertile week would shift to day 14 to 21.

We would recommend that a couple tries to conceive by making love every day or at least every other day over their fertile week. This is fine if you have a regular cycle, but what happens if yours is not regular and can vary in length from 26 days to 35 days? If your cycle changes all the time, you can't really predict your fertile week. To ensure you make love around the time of ovulation, you would have to start making love on day 8 of your next cycle and continue through to day 24, making love on every day or at least every other day. This can obviously put quite a strain on any relationship, and where couples have careers or work shifts it can become impossible.

If you want to conceive but your cycle is irregular and you are not willing to wait one or two years before looking for help, what can you do to help yourself?

The first thing to remember is that infertility is not just a woman's problem. It can only really be a problem for a couple. So, trying to help yourself means working together as a couple. Of those couples who go to infertility clinics, roughly speaking one-third of the problems are of female origin, one-third are of male, and one third are combined problems or no obvious problem can be identified. When looking at the female causes, about half of them are due to a failure to ovulate.

We know that conceiving and pregnancy outcomes are improved by the improved health of both partners. There are many studies now demonstrating that the better the health of both partners, the more likely is conception, the less likely are genetic and chromosomal defects, and the better a chance that the pregnancy will proceed normally. Even if you have a problem with ovulating which eventually needs medical treatment, the better your health and that of your partner, the better the outcome is likely to be.

Again, weight management is very important for women with PCOS, and an infertile woman with PCOS who is not ovulating may begin to ovulate again if she loses even just 5 per cent of her body weight.

The four-point plan outlined in Chapter 10 should be the first step in starting to help yourself and your partner. It will take several months to have an effect, in part because sperm production takes 120 days. We would recommend when planning to have a baby that preconceptual care should commence about six months before you actually want to start trying to conceive.

Tests for Infertility

A man will be asked to produce a sperm sample. A normal sperm count is above 20 million sperm per millilitre, and a good count is greater than 60 million per ml. Not all the sperms will be normal. The abnormal ones are counted and should be less than half. Similarly, more than half should be swimming normally. A poor sperm count with a high number of abnormal forms and poor swimmers can all be improved with good exercise and nutrition while avoiding chemical toxins from alcohol and smoking.

The investigations for a woman would include confirming ovulation. This is done by blood tests looking for the rise of progesterone in the second half of the menstrual cycle. If ovulation cannot be confirmed in this way then it is possible to have a number of ultrasound scans to follow the hopeful growth of the follicle during the first half of the cycle.

If you are not ovulating, besides weight reduction if this is needed, treatment options that your doctor or gynaecologist can offer are outlined in Chapter 8. Ovulation can also be encouraged using drugs such as clomiphene, or in some cases an operation called ovarian diathermy.

Once ovulation has been confirmed, the next check would be to confirm that the uterus and tubes are normal and free to transport the eggs after ovulation. This is done often by an operation called a laparoscopy.

During a laparoscopy, while you are under general anaesthetic a small telescope is inserted into your abdomen to allow the doctors to see the pelvic organs. Then some dye can be passed through the vagina, cervix and uterus to check that none of the tubes or passages are blocked in any way. Past pelvic infections, particularly with the bug called chlamydia, are now most common cause of tubal damage.

The only other test that is commonly performed is a special X-ray that looks at the cavity of the womb, although alternatively this can by done using another telescope investigation at the same time as a laparoscopy. This is used to confirm that the inside of the womb is normal.

Tubal damage can sometimes be repaired. Even if it is severe, the tubes can be by-passed using IVF techniques.

For more information about infertility and the treatments that are available for it, please see the Further Reading and Useful Addresses chapters.

See also **Miscarriage**

INSOMNIA

See **Sleep Problems**

IRRITABILITY

Feeling as if everything in the world is out to annoy you can come as part and parcel of PMS, but some women with PCOS say they feel this way a lot of the time. Thankfully there are many simple self-help steps you can take to help relieve an irritable, tense mood.

Touch Is Soothing

Remember how relaxing it was to have your mother brush your hair when you were little? Research has shown that massage reduces stress and anxiety, so book yourself in for a session in your PMT week. Or spend just 10 minutes stroking your ears, rubbing your feet, brushing your hair, massaging your scalp (easy when you're washing your hair) or giving yourself a massage – always rub towards your heart, either in circles or long strokes. Getting someone else to do this for you is even better – they can get to parts that you can't reach, especially tension hot spots like the back of your neck and shoulders.

Stroke Your Pet

A recent Australian study showed that 79 per cent of pet owners felt better if they spent time with their pets in times of stress. Other research shows being near friendly pets or watching fish can actually lower blood pressure.

Try a Mini Meditation

Close your eyes and concentrate on the sound of your own breathing. This focus will make you breathe more deeply and take your mind away from anything that's annoying you. If you find your mind slipping back into your day-to-day worries, nudge it back into concentrating on your breath.

Flower Remedies

If you're really snappy and stressed, try a few drops of Bach Rescue Remedy on your tongue – it's the energy of flowers captured in brandy and lots of people swear by it.

Essential Oils

Geranium essential oil has been shown to help lift depression, lavender to help dissolve aggression by de-stressing you. Add 3 drops to a warm (not hot) bath or burner.

Walking

Go for a brisk walk. Fresh air and the feelgood factor that comes with exercise will help to restore your balance.

JOINT PAIN

Although this is not a generally accepted symptom of PCOS, some women do complain that it affects them in the run-up to a period or when the weather is damp. Good ways to ease aching joints include a hot water bottle, baths with a warming aromatherapy oil such as ginger or black pepper (use sparingly, as these can irritate sensitive skin), and gentle massage which can also incorporate warming essential oils.

Please note: It is always worth ruling out other conditions such as arthritis with your doctor if you have persistent pain in your joints.

MENTAL FOGGINESS

❊ *Around a week before my period I can't concentrate at work and my brain is like mush.* Andie, 26

A lot of women with PCOS find that mental clarity goes out of the window as their menstrual cycle progresses.

Taking up a gentle mind/body exercise such as yoga or tai chi can help to promote clearer thinking, as well as lowering stress levels and increasing fitness.

Food supplements such as gingko biloba and phosphetidyl serine have also been shown to improve short-term memory and increase blood flow to the brain to help encourage clearer thinking.

For a quick fix of clarity, try sucking on a mint or sniffing a tissue with a couple of drops of peppermint essential oil on it – this has been shown to help improve concentration and alertness, as has rosemary. Dab a couple of drops on a tissue and sniff it every 10 minutes or so.

Going for a walk around the block in the fresh air can also help to blow away the cobwebs and sharpen up your mind if you're having a bad brain day, as can making sure you have healthy snacks to hand, such as carrot sticks, a fruit muffin or a piece of fresh or dried fruit combined with a handful of nuts.

MISCARRIAGE

Miscarriage is the name given to the accidental or spontaneous loss of a developing foetus before 28 weeks. Around one in six confirmed pregnancies ends in miscarriage, many in the first 12 weeks. Women with PCOS, however, are at an increased risk of miscarriage.

The reasons for this are still unclear, says Professor Stephen Franks, who states

✿ *Miscarriage is more likely to occur in women with PCOS, though it was previously thought to be much more common than it is now believed to be. If you ovulate and conceive you can expect to have a normal pregnancy. It is unusual to have repeated miscarriage. Raised levels of the hormone known as LH, luteinizing hormone, are thought to be associated with this risk but at present it is unclear exactly what the link is.*

The other common explanation is that the foetus was not developing properly and therefore the womb shed it.

If you know you are pregnant and you experience period-like pains in your abdomen and lower back, or you notice bleeding (clots of a dark brown vaginal discharge), go to see a doctor or midwife immediately. If a miscarriage is suspected you will normally be offered an ultrasound scan. With this it is possible to identify if you have just had a small bleed and the pregnancy is still viable and will continue, or if the pregnancy has been lost.

After a miscarriage treatment can include a procedure known as a D & C, in which the womb lining is scraped away to avoid infection; or a course of antibiotics if an infection is suspected or has set in.

If you go through three or more miscarriages in a row you and your partner may be given a full check-up to make sure you have no latent infections in the reproductive organs.

You can also explore the option of preconceptual care where you both get yourselves up to peak physical and nutritional health before trying again for a baby. Always check if your doctor or hospital will refer you for this treatment. Otherwise, contact a nutritional therapist with a good track record in this area, or contact an organization devoted to pre-conceptual care (see the Useful Addresses chapter).

However, the emotional toll of a miscarriage is often the most difficult aspect to deal with. Your doctor should be able to refer you, your partner if you have one, or the two of you as a couple to a trained counsellor who can help you come to terms with your emotions and your loss. Support from friends and family is also important – don't be afraid to ask for it, as some people can be embarrassed about mentioning it to you because they don't want to make you more upset. You can also contact support groups to share your feelings with other people who have been through a similar thing and know something of how you feel.

For general emotional and physical healing, and to help restore your relationship with your body, complementary therapies such as aromatherapy massage, energy/spiritual healing and homoeopathy can all be helpful. Bach Flower Remedies which may help include Star of Bethlehem for shock, and Gentian for distress.

MOOD SWINGS

Vitamin B_6 is the classic remedy for mood swings related to PMS or hormonal disturbance, and is available on prescription or over the counter. A magnesium supplement can also be helpful. Dr Maryon Stewart, who founded and runs the Women's Nutritional Advisory Service, says between 50 and 80 per cent of the women consulting the WNAS due to PMS or menopausal changes including mood swings were found to be deficient in magnesium.

Exercise such as a brisk walk can help to lift a low mood. (See also our mood-lifting ideas in the section on Depression, above.)

If your mood swings make you feel out of control and a bit disoriented, simple breathing exercises can be grounding. Try closing your eyes and taking 10 breaths as deeply into your body as you can. Hold for 5 seconds before releasing. Or try reversing your breathing cycle, so that instead of making an effort to breathe in, you make an effort to breathe out and let the in-breath happen by itself. The easiest way to do this is simply to force out as much air as you can from your lungs on an out-breath and go from here. It sounds odd, but it is calming.

The following aromatherapy oils are also good to help bring a sense of balance and solidity to your emotional state: bergamot, camomile, clary sage, geranium, frankincense, juniper, lavender, rosewood, sage, sandalwood, vetivert and ylang ylang. Choose the one you like the best (this may vary from day to day), adding a couple of drops to a tissue, a burner or your bath.

NAUSEA

In the same way that fluctuating hormones during pregnancy can lead to feelings of nausea, some women with PCOS find that they feel sick around the middle of a menstrual cycle (however long that may be), before a period or during one. Eating light foods, drinking peppermint tea and eating an apple can all help to alleviate nausea, as can the spice ginger, which has been shown in studies to reduce feelings of sickness significantly. Chew on a chocolate ginger, a piece of crystallized ginger, eat a light stir-fry with ginger seasoning or take ginger supplements, available from most pharmacies.

Also be aware that nausea can come on if you haven't eaten properly, as well as, of course, with illnesses such as a cold, flu or food poisoning.

OBESITY

If you are 3 stone (42 lb/19 kg) overweight, then losing the ideal 1 or 2 pounds each week will mean that it should take at least six months to get to your ideal body weight. If you lose weight faster than this it is likely you will probably be losing muscle mass. This will be detrimental in the long term, as a loss of muscle mass will further reduce your metabolic weight, making it difficult to stay at your new weight and making further weight loss even harder.

The good news is that once you start, even small weight losses will be associated with noticeable changes in symptoms. You will not have to wait to reach your ideal weight before you start to feel the benefits. Research has shown that with as little as a 5 per cent reduction in body weight women with PCOS and irregular periods and infertility saw an

82 per cent improvement in their symptoms and developed a regular menstrual cycle or conceived. There was also a 40 per cent improvement in hirsutism.[3] This means if you were now 12 stone (168 lb/76 kg) you could expect to see an improvement of symptoms after losing only just over half a stone (8 lb/3.8 kg).

Although the incidence of obesity in women with PCOS is actually not much different to that of the general population, the implications of weight gain for women with PCOS are different, with research by Professor Stephen Franks at St Mary's Hospital in London showing a higher proportion of overweight women with PCOS having unwanted hair and irregular or non-existent periods. Leaner women had fewer symptoms. So putting on more weight is one of the triggers for making symptoms worse, or even for pushing a woman with PCO into having PCOS.

Putting on more weight if you have PCOS can also increase your chances of developing diabetes. Losing even 5 to 10 per cent of your body weight can dramatically improve symptoms as well as helping to safeguard against diabetes.

In theory this should be fairly straightforward, but many women with PCOS find that not only do they gain weight easily, but they also find it very difficult to lose it once it's there. A woman with PCOS is now believed to have a different metabolism to that of a woman without PCOS, in that she burns calories at a different rate and stores fat more efficiently, thus making it harder to lose weight once it has been put on.

Your Questions Answered

Can Weight Loss Drugs Help?
The weight loss drugs that interfere with fat absorption cannot be recommended as a strategy for weight management.

Does Metformin Work as a Weight Loss Tool?

There is some new work suggesting that Metformin may be useful as part of weight management program. It improves insulin sensitivity and this encourages weight loss. This will be further improved when combined with an exercise program. There may be a role for its use in the future to start the process of weight loss off and improve insulin sensitivity, with the hope that once a person is again slim and fit they would not need to continue with the treatment.

Does Coming Off the Pill Help?

The decision to come off the Pill is complicated and needs to be addressed on an individual basis with your doctor. For women who have used the Pill to regulate their cycle, coming off the Pill may mean that they have few or no periods.

Practical Steps for Losing Weight

Changing eating patterns and following the four-point plan outlined in Chapter 10 can help to control PCOS and help you lose weight at the same time. We all know what basic healthy eating and exercise involves – less fat, less sugar and more exercise are the three basic steps that most of us know we should take to improve our health, whether we have PCOS or not. If you need help and ideas to get started on a healthy eating program, talk to your doctor. He or she may be able to recommend a dietitian or nutritionist. You could also contact a nutritional therapist. Or have a look in your local bookstore for low-fat, low-sugar recipe books that look inviting – also see the Further Reading chapter.

Controlling your snacking is another good way to stop weight creeping on. Eating five small meals a day to keep blood sugar levels constant can help, but this is sometimes just not practical. See the section on Food Cravings, above, for some tips on healthy snacks to eat at home and at work.

Support from other people is useful when you are trying to lose weight. Losing weight is a complex issue and difficult for most of the population, not just women with PCOS – that's why you can join weight loss clubs, or ask your doctor to refer you to a clinic where your weight loss can be monitored regularly. Getting your friends, colleagues and family to support you can also be a great help – if they understand you are trying to lose weight they are less likely to pressure you to have dessert or another drink, etc.

PERIOD PAIN

Period pain can be debilitating and draining, making the day much harder to cope with. There are many over-the-counter painkillers to use, but there are also an increasing number of natural painkillers around.

- ❋ TENS machines are small units which you can attach to your abdomen. They use mild electronic pulses to scramble the nerves' pain signals to the brain. They are available from pharmacies and many major stores.
- ❋ The good old hot water bottle.
- ❋ A warm bath with a couple of drops of geranium (mood-lifting), camomile (painkilling) and clary sage (muscle-relaxant) oils can help to ease cramping and soothe pain.
- ❋ Gentle exercise can help to relieve menstrual cramps. Wrap yourself up in a cozy sweater and go for a stroll around the block. You'll be surprised at the results.
- ❋ Willow bark and kava kava tablets are the natural alternatives to aspirin, available from healthfood stores and herbalists.

SLEEP PROBLEMS

Many women experience lighter sleep, difficulty getting to sleep or disturbances such as waking in the night just before and during a period. Some women with PCOS find their sleep is constantly disrupted. This could be due to hormonal fluctuations, which should be helped as you begin treatment for PCOS.

However, some emotional factors such as anxiety or stress can also contribute. Although these can be caused by having to deal with PCOS and the issues surrounding it, they can also be caused by life in general. Trying to identify the causes of stress, anxiety and worry of any kind is therefore the first step towards improving sleep quality. If it turns out to be work, money or a family issue, for example, sorting this out could help enormously.

The environment in which you sleep can also have a profound effect on your quality of rest. Make sure your bedroom isn't noisy, too light, too crammed with untidy piles of stuff, too hot or too cold. Try not to watch TV in bed, or to drink coffee or smoke before you try and sleep, as these are stimulants which activate your brain and excite your body into thinking it should stay awake.

Lack of exercise can also lead to restlessness as your body still hasn't worked off the energy it has received from the food you have eaten during the day. Don't exercise just before bed, as this also wakes up your body and brain and can stop you sleeping.

Home Help for Better Sleep

❋ Lavender essential oil is famous for its soothing and relaxing qualities. Sprinkle a couple of drops on your pillow or in a warm bedtime bath to help you unwind.

❋ Having a hot water bottle for your feet can help you sleep more soundly, according to research recently published in *Nature* magazine. Feet are warmer when you are in deep sleep, and speeding up the heating process can trick you into sleeping more deeply more quickly.

❋ Use your imagination. Allow your mind to drift off into a happy memory, for example, or imagine yourself on a warm beach, listening to the shush of the sea, smelling the suntan oil and enjoying the warmth. This will help you to relax and even encourage you to drift off into sleep.

❋ Herbal and homoeopathic 'sleeping pills' can help you to get a good rest without giving you the hangover effect of traditional sleeping pills. Pharmacies and herbalists sell these – look for the herbs valerian, hops and passiflora.

❀ Spend 10 minutes lying in bed and listening to the sound of your own deep breathing, as this can help to relax you and take your mind off the fact that you are trying hard to get to sleep.

References

CHAPTER I: PCOS? NEVER HEARD OF IT!

1 Polson, D W, Adams, J, Wadsworth, J and Franks, S 'Polycystic ovaries –
a common finding in normal women', Lancet i (1988): 870–2
2 Franks, S 'Polycystic ovary syndrome', Engl J Med 333 (1995): 853–61

CHAPTER 2: WHAT IS POLYCYSTIC OVARY SYNDROME?

1 Stein, I F and Leventhal, M L 'Amenorrhea associated with bilateral
polycystic ovaries', Am J Obstet Gynecol 29 (1935):181–91
2 Adams, J, Franks, S, Polson, D W et al, 'Multifollicular ovaries: Clinical and
endocrine feature and response to pulsatile gonadotrophin releasing
hormone', Lancet ii (1985): 1375–78
3 Adams, J, Polson D W and Franks, S 'Prevalence of polycystic ovaries in
women with anovulation and idiopathic hirsutism', Br Med J 293 (1986):355–9
4 Polson, D W, Adams, J, Wadsworth, J and Franks, S 'Polycystic ovaries – a
common finding in normal women', Lancet i (1988):870–2
5 Gilling-Smith, C and Franks, S 'Polycystic ovary syndrome', Repord Med Rev 2
(1993): 15–32
6 Green, J A and Goldzeiher, J W 'The polycystic ovary. Light and electron
microscope studies', Am J Obstet Gynecol 91 (1965):173–81
7 Conway, G S, Honour, J W and Jacobs, H S 'Heterogeneity of the polycystic
ovary syndrome: clinical, endocrine and ultrasound features in 556 patients',
Clin Endocrinol (Oxf) 30 (1989):459–70

CHAPTER 4: WHAT CAUSES PCOS?

1 Jacobs, H S The LH hypotheses, in Shaw, R W (ed.) Advances in Reproductive
Endocrinology: Polycystic Ovaries – A Disorder or a Symptom? The Parthenon
Publishing Group (1991):91–8
2 Regan, L, Owen, E and Jacobs, H S 'Hypersecretion of LH, infertility and
spontaneous abortion', Lancet 336 (8724) (1990):1141–44
3 Franks, S 'The ubiquitous polycystic ovary', J of Endocrinol 129 (1991):317–19
4 Barnes, R B, Rosenfield, R L, Bursyein, S and Ehrmann, D A 'Pituitary-
ovarain response to nafarelin testing in polycystic ovary syndrome', N Engl J
Med 320 (1989):559–65
5 Rosenfield, R L, Barnes, R B, Cara, J F and Lucky, A W 'Dysregulation of
cytochrome P450c 17 alpha as the cause of polycystic ovarian syndrome',
Fertility and Sterility 53 (1990):785–91
6 Ehrmann, D A, Rosenfield, R L, Barnes, R B, Brigell, D F and Sheikh, Z
'Detection of functional ovarian hyperandrogenism in women with androgen
excess', N Engl J Med 337 (1992):157–62

7 Carey, A H, Chan, K L, Short, F, White, D M, Williamson, R and Franks, S 'Evidence for a single gene effect in polycystic ovaries and premature male pattern baldness', *Clin Endocrinol* 38 (1993):653–8
8 Carey, A H, Waterworth, D, Patel, K, White, D, Little, J, Novelli, P, Franks, S and Williamson, R 'Polycystic ovaries and premature male pattern baldness are associated with one allele of the steroid metabolism gene CYP17', *Human Molecular Genetics* 3 (1994):1873–76
9 Gharani, N, Waterworth, D M, Williamson, R and Franks, S '5'polymorphism of the CYP17 gene is not associated with serum testosterone levels in women with polycystic ovaries', *J Clin Endocrin* 81 (1996):4147
10 Burghen, G A, Givens, J R and Kitabchi, A E 'Correlation of hyperandrogenism with hyperinsulinism and polycystic ovarian disease', *J Clin Endocrinol Metab* 50 (1980):113–16
11 Chang, R J, Nakamura, R M, Judd, H L and Kaplan, S A 'Insulin resistance in non-obese patients with polycystic ovarian disease', *J Clin Endocrinol Metab* 57 (1983):356–9
12 Barbieri, R L and Horstein, M D 'Hyperinsulinemia and ovarian hyperandrogenism', *Endocrinol Metab Clinics N Am* 17 (1988):685–703
13 Franks, S, Gharani, N, Waterworth, D M, Batty, S, White, D, Williamson, R and McCarthy, M 'The genetic basis of polycystic ovary syndrome', *Human Reproduction* 12 (1997):2641–48
14 Gharani, N, Waterworth, D M, Batty, S, White, D, Gilling-Smith, C, Conway, G S, McCarthy M, Franks, S and Williamson, R 'Association of the steroid metabolising gene CPY11a with polycystic ovary syndrome and hyperandrogenism', *Human Molecular Genetics* 6 (1997):397–402
15 Waterworth, D M, Bennett, S T, Gharani, N, McCarthy, M, Hague, S, Batty, S, Conway, G S, White, D, Todd, J A, Franks, S and Williamson, R 'Linkage and association of insulin gene VNTR regulatory polymorphism with polycystic ovary syndrome', *Lancet* 349 (1997):1771–72
16 Dahlgren, E, Johansson, S, Lindstedt, G et al 'Women with polycystic ovary syndrome wedge resection in 1956 to 1965: a long term follow-up on natural history and circulation hormones', *Fertility and Sterility* 57 (1992):505–13

CHAPTER 5: HOW OUR LIFESTYLE AFFECTS PCOS

1 Hall, R H 'The agri-business view of soil and life', *J Holistic Med.* 3 (1981): 157–66
2 Rose, E F 'The effects of soil and diet on disease', *Cancer Res.* 28 (1968): 2390–2
3 Schroeder, H A 'Losses of vitamins and trace minerals resulting from processing and preservation of foods', *Am J Clin Nutr.* 24 (1971): 562–73
4 Morris, B 'Correlations between abnormalities in chromium and glucose metabolism in a group of diabetics', *Clin Chem* 34 (1988): 1525–26
5 Davies, S 'Age-related decreases in chromium in 51,665 hair, sweat and serum samples from 40,872 patients – implications for the prevention of cardiovascular disease and type II diabetes mellitus', *Metabolism* 46.5 (1997): 1–4

6 Abrahamns, A S 'The effect of chromium supplementation on serum glucose and lipids in patients with and without non-insulin-dependant diabetes', *Metabolism* 41 (1992): 768

7 Railes, R 'Effect of chromium chloride supplementation in glucose tolerance and serum lipids including high density lipoproteins of adult men', *Am J Clin Nutr* 34 (1981): 2670–8

8 Anderson, R A, Cheng, N, Bryden, N A *et al* 'Elevated intakes of supplemental chromium improves glucose and insulin variables in individuals with type 2 diabetes', *Diabetes* 47 (1997): 1786–91

9 Kirksey, A *et al* 'Vitamin status of a group of female adolescents', *Am J Clin Nutr.* 31 (1978): 946–54; Guilland, J C *et al* 'Evaluation of pyridoxine intake and pyridoxine status among aged institutionalized people', *Int J Vitam Nutr Res.* 54 (1984): 185–93

10 Chappell, L C, Seed, P T, Briley, A L *et al* 'Effect of antioxidants on the occurrence of pre-eclampsia in women at increased risk: a randomised trial', *Lancet* 354 (1999):788–9

11 National Research Council, Food and Nutrition Board *Toward Healthful Diets* (Washington, DC: Academy of Sciences, 1980)

12 Reilly, J J, Dorosty, A R and Emmett, P M 'Prevalence of overweight and obesity in British children', *BMJ* 319 (1999): 1039

CHAPTER 6: LONG-TERM HEALTH CONSEQUENCES

1 Evans, D J, Hoffman, D G, Kalkhoff, R K and Kissebah, A H 'Relationship of androgenic activity to body fat topography, fat cell morphology and metabolic aberrations in premenopausal women', *J Clin Endocrinol Metab* 57 (1983):304–10

2 Wild, R A, Painter, P C, Coulson, P B *et al* 'Lipoprotein lipid concentrations and cardiovascular risk in women with polycystic ovary syndrome', *J Clin Endocrinol Metab* 61 (1985):946–51

3 Conway, G S, Agrawal, R, Betteridge, D J *et al* 'Risk factors for coronary artery disease in lean and obese women with polycystic ovary syndrome', *J Clin Endocrinol* 37 (1992):119–25

4 Dahlgreen, E, Johansson, S, Lindstedt, G *et al* 'Women with polycystic ovary syndrome wedge resection in 1956 to 1965: a long term follow-up on natural history and circulation hormones', *Fertility and Sterility* 57 (1992):505–13

5 Gjonaess, H 'The course and outcome of pregnancy after ovarian electrocautery in women with polycystic ovary syndrome: the influence of body weight', *Br J Obstet Gynaecol* 98 (1989):714–19

6 Dahlgreen, E, Johansson, S, Lindstedt, G *et al* 'Women with polycystic ovary syndrome wedge resection in 1956 to 1965: a long term follow-up on natural history and circulation hormones', *Fertility and Sterility* 57 (1992):505–13

7 Dahlgreen, E, Janson, P O, Johansson, S, Lapidus, L and Oden, A 'Polycystic ovary syndrome and risk for myocardial infarction: evaluation from a risk factor model based on a prospective study of women', *Acta Obstet Gynecol Scand* 71 (1992):119–25

8 Rajkhowa, M, Glass, M R, Rutherford, A J, Michelmore, K and Balen, A H 'Polycystic ovary syndrome: a risk factor for cardiovascular disease?' *Br J Obstet Gynaecol* 10 (2000):11–18

CHAPTER 12: A–Z OF SYMPTOMS

1 Goldstein, Dr S R and Ashner, L *Could It Be the Perimenopause?* (Vermilion, 1999)
2 Study published in *Archives of Dermatology*, December 1998
3 Kiddy, D S, Hamilton-Fairley, D, Bush, A *et al* 'Improvement in endocrine and ovarian function during dietary treatment of obese women with polycystic ovary syndrome', *Clinical Endocrinology* 36 (1992): 105–11

Further Reading

UK buyers in the US can buy the US titles listed from Airlift Books: mail order on 0181 804 0400.

ACNE

Aloe Vera, Julia Lawless and Judith Allen (Thorsons)
Good Skin Doctor, Anne Lovell and Tony Chu (Thorsons)
Natural Skincare (Frog Limited, available from Airlift)

BODY IMAGE

Beauty Wisdom/Simply Radiant, Bharti Vyas (Thorsons)
Body Image Workbook (New Harbinger Publications, available from Airlift)
How You Feel Is Up to You (Impact, available from Airlift)
Self-esteem, Gael Lindenfield (Thorsons)
Self-esteem Companion (New Harbinger, available from Airlift)
Self-esteem – A Proven Programme (New Harbinger, available from Airlift)
611 Ways to Boost Your Self-esteem (Health Communications, available from Airlift)
Transforming Body Image (Crossing, available from Airlift)
200 Ways to Love the Body You Have (Crossing Press, available from Airlift)

COMPLEMENTARY THERAPIES

Bach Flower Therapy, Mechthild Schiffer (Thorsons)
The Element Encyclopaedias of Herbalism, Homoeopathy, Aromatherapy, Reflexology, Ayurveda, Massage (Element Books)
The Fragrant Mind, *The Fragrant Pharmacy* and *The Fragrant Heavens*, Valerie Ann Worwood (Doubleday)
The Hamlyn Encyclopaedia of Complementary Therapies – an amazingly informative and useful book
Herbal Defence, Robyn Landis with Karta Purkh Singh Khalsan (Thorsons)
Woman Medicine – Vitex Agnus Castus, Simon Mills (Amberwood Publishing) and *Vitex – the Women's Herb* by Christopher Hobbs (Botanica)
Holistic Woman's Herbal, Kitty Campion (Bloomsbury)
Women's Encyclopaedia of Natural Medicine (Keats, available from Airlift)

DEPRESSION

Burned Out and Blue, Kristina Downing Orr (Thorsons)
Depression – with information on conventional and alternative approaches (Element's Natural Way series)
St John's Wort: Your Natural Prozac, Dr Norman Rosenthal (Thorsons)

DETOX

Cleanse Your System, Amanda Ursell (Thorsons)
Detoxification and Healing (Keats, available from Airlift)
Natural Detox, Marie Farquharson (Element)

DIABETES

Coping with Diabetes (Avery, available from Airlift)
Diabetes – with information on conventional and alternative approaches (Element's Natural Way series)
The Diabetes Cure, Vern S Cherewatenko and Paul Perry (Thorsons) – about Type II diabetes
Healthy Living with Diabetes (New Harbinger, available from Airlift)
Vegetarian Cookbook for people with diabetes (Book Publishing Co, available from Airlift)
Victory over Diabetes (Keats, available from Airlift)

FATIGUE

Thyroid – Why am I so Tired?, Martin Budd (Thorsons)

HAIR LOSS

The Hair Loss Cure – Elizabeth Steele (founder of the self help group Hairline International) (Thorsons)

HEALTHY EATING

Healing with Wholefoods (North Atlantic, available from Airlift)
The Optimum Nutrition Cookbook, Patrick Holford and Judy Ridgway (Piatkus)
The Sunday Times Vitality Cookbook, Susan Clark (HarperCollins)

HEALTHY LIVING

8 Weeks to Optimum Health, Andrew Weil (Littlebrown)
Women's Bodies, Women's Wisdom, Dr Christiane Northrup (Piatkus)

INFERTILITY

The Infertility Book (Celestial, available from Airlift)
The Infertility Companion, Anna Furse (Thorsons)
Infertility – the last secret (what happens when you want to have a baby), Anna McGrail (Bloomsbury)
Infertility – a sympathetic approach to understanding the causes and options for treatment, Professor Robert Winston (Vermilion)

SEX

The Art of Sexual Ecstasy, Margo Anand (Jeremy P. Tarcher)
The Cosmopolitan Guide to love, sex and relationships by Philip Hodson (Headline)
The Dating Game – Guerrilla Dating Tactics! Sharyn Wolf (Thorsons) – good for those who want funny advice on the dating scene
Hot Monogamy Dr Patricia Love and Jo Robinson (Piatkus)
Increase Your Sex Drive, Dr Sarah Brewer (Thorsons) – also has a lot about making you feel confident sexually

STRESS

101 Shortcuts to relaxation by Cathy Hopkins (Bloomsbury)
The New Life Library – instant Calm, Natural Ways to reduce stress (Lorenz Books)
Stressbusters, Robert Holden (Thorsons)
Timeshifting, Stephen Rechstaffen (Vermilion)

Useful Addresses

This is a list of places where you can find out more about PCOS in general, your specific symptoms and therapies you may choose to help you deal with it both physically and emotionally. Always send a stamped addressed envelope if you write off somewhere, as many of these places are charities or run by volunteers.

The Internet can also be a huge source of information and support. Many libraries have the facility for you to use a computer to surf the Net, as do some cybercafes in many towns and cities.

The publishers have checked addresses and phone numbers at the time of going to press, but cannot be responsible for associations that have changed their contact addresses since that time.

UK

PCOS SUPPORT AND INFORMATION
VERITY
52–54 Featherstone Street
London EC1Y 8RT

ACNE
Acne Support Group
PO Box 230
Hayes
Middlesex UB4 0UT
www.m2w3.com/acne
020 8561 6868
www.healthy.net/LIBRARY/BOOKS/Healthyself.acne.htm
The Sher System
Acne helpline: 020 7499 4022

ALOPECIA
Hairline International – The Alopecia Patients Society
Lyons Court
1668 High Street
Knowle
West Midlands B93 0LY
01564 775281

Alopecia website
http://follicle.com/types.html

COUNSELLING
British Association for Counselling
1 Regent Place
Rugby
Warwickshire CV21 2PJ
01788 550899

DEPRESSION
Depression Alliance
35 Westminster Bridge Road
London SE1 7JB
020 7633 9929

DIABETES
British Diabetic Association
10 Queen Anne Street
London W1M 0BD
020 7323 1531

EATING DISORDERS
Tottenham Women's Health Centre
15 Fenhurst Gate
Aughton
Ormskirk
Lancs L39 5ED
01695 422 479
Eating Disorders Association
Sackville Place
44 Magdalen Street
Norwich
Norfolk NR3 1JE
01603 621 414
Eating Disorder Recovery
1-888-520-1700
email: jrust@edrecovery.com
www.edrecovery.com/
Eating Disorder Support (online)
http://www.anorexia.org/chat/

ENDOMETRIOSIS
The SHE Trust
Simply Holistic Endometriosis
Red Hall Lodge
Red Hall Drive
Bracebridge Heath
Lincoln LN4 2JT
www.endometriosis.co.uk
www.shetrust.org.uk

EXCESS HAIR
Epilight
For an information pack telephone 07000 560821
British Association of Electrolysis
01895 239966
Institute of Electrolysis
01908 695297

FERTILITY AND PRE-CONCEPTUAL CARE
National Childbirth Trust
Alexandra House
Oldham Terrace
Acton
London W3 7NH
Foresight Association for the Promotion of Pre-Conceptual Care
28 The Paddock
Goldalming
Surrey GU7 1XD
01483 427 839
Issue – Infertility Support
509 Aldridge Road
Great Barr
Birmingham B44
0121 344 4414
0121 344 4336
www.ein.org

HEALTHY EATING
Organic Growers Association
Aeron Park
Llangietho
Dyfed
Wales

Soil Association
86 Colston Street
Bristol BS1 5BB UK
Freshwater Filters
Carlton House
Aylmer Road
Leystone E11 3AD
Friends of the Earth
26–28 Underwood Street
London N1 7JQ

MISCARRIAGE
Miscarriage Association
c/o Clayton Hospital
Northgate
Wakefield
W Yorks WF1 3JS
01924 200 799
Useful Websites
Why did I have a miscarriage?
www.womens-health.co.uk/miscarr.htm
Infertility and miscarriage research studies
www.chem-tox.com/infertility
Support groups listings
www.kumc.edu/gec/support/miscarri.html
Practical tips on coping after pregnancy loss
web.co.nz/~katef/sspl/
Fears about subsequent pregnacy
www.townonline.com/marblehead/entertainment/health/028985 2 pregnancy
Miscarriage chat room
chat.hcc.cc.fl.us/dbgchat1.html

NUTRITION
British Association of Nutritional Therapists
PO Box 17436
London SE13 7WT
The Centre for Nutritional Medicine
114 Harley Street
London W1N 1AG
020 7224 5053
www.2xlnutrition.com
Women's Nutritional Advisory Service
01273 487366
Can help you change your diet to help get your body back on track

ALTERNATIVE THERAPIES
Institute for Complementary Medicine
PO Box 194
London SE16 1QZ
020 7237 5165
British Complementary Medicine Association
249 Fosse Rd
Leicester LE3 1AE
0116 282 5511
Register of Chinese Herbal Medicine
PO Box 400
Middlesex HA9 9NZ
020 7224 0883
British Acupuncture Council
Park House
206–208 Latimer Road
London W10 6RE
020 8964 0222
The Society of Teachers of Alexander Technique
20 London House
266 Fulham Road
London SW10 9EL
020 7351 0828
Aromatherapy Organizations Council
PO Box 355
Croydon CR9 2QP
020 8251 7912
Frances Box, Aromatherapist and Reflexologist
Ceres Natural Health and Beauty
01306 627703
The Bach Centre (Bach Flower Remedies)
Mount Vernon
Sotwell
Wallingford
Oxfordshire OX10 0PZ
01491 834678
The Colour Therapy Association
PO Box 16756
London SW20 8ZW
020 8540 3540
National Federation of Spiritual Healers
0891 616080 (48p/min peak rate, Mon- Fri), or send A5 sae to:
Old Manor Farm Studio
Church Street
Sunbury-on-Thames
Middlesex TW16 6RG

General Council and Register of Consultant Herbalists
32 King Edwards Road
Swansea SA1 4LL
01792 655886 (9 a.m.–2 p.m. Mon-Fri)
National Institute of Medical Herbalists
56 Longbrook Street
Exeter
Devon EX4 6AH
01392 426022
Fiona Waller, Medical Herbalist
Clissold Park Natural Health Centre
London
Society of Homoeopaths
2 Artizan Road
Northampton NN1 4HU
01604 621400
British Homeopathic Association
27a Devonshire Street
London W1N 1RJ
020 7935 2163
Moira Houston, Registered Homoeopath
The Chatsworth Clinic
Kilburn, London
020 8451 4754
Letchworth Centre
Hertfordshire
01462 678804
British Society for Medical and Dental Hypnosis
151 Otley Old Road
Leeds LS16 6HN
Laughter Therapy
In the UK, proof of a good giggle's restorative powers helped persuade the NHS to set up a laughter clinic run by Robert Holden:
The Happiness Project
01865 244414
The London College of Massage and Shiatsu
21 Portland Place
London W1N 3AF
The Academy of On-site Massage
01453 521530
The Vital Touch
020 7431 8694
Heather Wood
020 8406 9182
The Mobile Feelgood Company
0800 731 5100

Camilla Ghazala
Indian head massage
01638 552047
Transcendental Meditation Association
Freepost London SW1P 4YY
0990 143733
General Council and Register of Naturopaths
Goswell House
2 Goswell Road
Street
Somerset BA16 0JG
01458 840072
Association of Reflexologists
27 Old Gloucester Street
London WC1N 3XX
08705 673320
Mel Jones, Registered Reflexologist
Cornbrook Bridge House
Clee Hill
Ludlow
Shropshire SY8 3QQ
01981 550829 (10 a.m.–2 p.m. weekdays)
The Shiatsu Society
Barber House
Storeys Bar Road
Sengate
Peterborough PE1 5YS
01733 758341
Yoga for Health Foundation
Ickwell Bury
Biggleswade
Bedfordshire SG18 9EF
01767 627271

USA

PCOS SUPPORT AND INFORMATION
Polycystic Ovarian Syndrome Association Inc
PO Box 80517
Portland, OR 97280
www.pcosupport.org
National Organization for Rare Disorders (US)
PO Box 8923
New Fairfield, CT 06812—8923
(203) 746-6518/(800) 999-6673
email: orphan@nord-rdb.com

www.nord-rdb.com/-orphan
(Despite PCOS being so common, this organization deals with it under the
name Stein Levanthal Syndrome)
www.soulcysters.com
Online support and a place to share PCOS histories

ACNE
Acne Network of America
members.tripod.com/~wildsurvival/index.html
www.stopspot.net (for teenagers dealing with acne)

ALOPECIA
Alopecia Support Group
Frank Smith
4488 Poplar Avenue
Dunnam 329
Memphis TN 381177
(901) 682-1103/(901) 761-0576
www.jericho.org/-jericho/_ccc_asg.html
Alopecia website
http://follicle.com/types.html

COUNSELLING
Concerned Counseling
Telephone counseling service toll-free within the US on 1-888-415-8255
http://concernedcounseling.com

DEPRESSION
National Institute of Mental Health
NIMH Public Inquiries
6001 Executive Boulevard
Rm 8184
MSC 9663
Bethesda MD 20892—9663
(301) 443-4513
Fax (301) 443-4279
www.nimh.nih.gov

DIABETES
The American Diabetes Association
www.diabetes.org
There's also an amazing website which links you to every other useful site on
diabetes:
www.mendosa.com/org.htm

EATING DISORDERS
Eating Disorder Recovery
1-888-520-1700
email: jrust@edrecovery.com
www.edrecovery.com
Eating Disorder Support (online)
www.anorexia.org/chat

ENDOMETRIOSIS
International Endometriosis Association
8585 N. 76th Place
Milwaukee WI 53223—2600
(800) 992-3636
Tel (414) 355 2200
Fax (414) 355-6065
www.endometriosisassn.org

FERTILITY AND PRE-CONCEPTUAL CARE
Infertility Network Exchange
PO Box 204
East Meadow, NY 11554
(516) 794-9772
The Fertility Institute
6020 Bullard Avenue
New Orleans, LA 70128
800 433-9009
www.fertilityinstitute.com
Information and support websites
www.4fertility.com/
alt.infertility.alternatives
www.preconception.com
www.obgyn.net

HEALTHY EATING
Center for Science in the Public Interest
Americans for Safe Food
1501 16th St, NW
Washington DC 20036
(202) 332-9110

MISCARRIAGE
Useful Websites
Why did I have a miscarriage?
www.womens-health.co.uk/miscarr.htm
Infertility and miscarriage research studies
www.chem-tox.com/infertility

Support groups listings
www.kumc.edu/gec/support/miscarri.html
Practical tips on coping after pregnancy loss
web.co.nz/~katef/sspl/
Fears about subsequent pregnancy
www.townonline.com/marblehead/entertainment/health
Miscarriage chat room
chat.hcc.cc.fl.us/dbgchat1.html

ALTERNATIVE THERAPIES
The American Association of Acupuncture and Oriental Medicine
433 Front Street
Catasauqua, PA 18032
North American Society of the Teachers of Alexander Technique
PO Box 517
Urbana, IL 61801—0517
(800) 473-0620
The American Alliance of Aromatherapy
PO Box 750428
Petalumo, CA 94975
Dr Edward Bach Healing Society
644 Merrick Road
Lynbrook, NY 11563
(516) 593-2206
College of Sytonic Optometry
1200 Robeson Street
Fall River, MA 02720—5308
(609) 692-4686
Spiritual Healing Common Boundary Inc
7005 Florida Street
Chevy Chase, MD 20815
The American Herbalist Guild
PO Box 1683
Sequel, CA 95073
North American Herbalists Guild
PO Box 1683
Sequel, CA 95073
American Foundation for Homeopathy
1508 S. Garfield
Alhambra, CA 91801
The Society for Clinical and Experimental Hypnosis
University of Colorado Medical Center
CO
American Massage Therapy Association
820 Davis Street
Suite 100
Evanston, IL 60210
(312) 761-2682

American Association of Naturopathic Physicians
PO Box 20386
Seattle, WA 98102
1-206-323-7610
American College of Advancement in Medicine
PO Box 3427
Laguna Hils, CA 92634
(714) 583-7666
International Institute of Reflexology
PO Box 12462
St Petersburg, FL 33733
(813) 343-4811
American Shiatsu Association
PO Box 718
Jamaica Plain, MA 01230
The American Yoga Association
513 South Orange Avenue
Sarasota, FL 34236
email: AmYogaAssn@aol.com.

CANADA

ALTERNATIVE THERAPIES
Canadian Naturopathic Association
205, 1234 17th Avenue South West
PO Box 3143
Station C
Calgary, Alberta
1-413-244-4487
Canadian Holistic Medical Association
491 Eglington Avenue West
Apt 407
Toronto, Ontario M5N 1A8
1-416-485-3071

AUSTRALIA

PCOS SUPPORT AND INFORMATION
Polycystic Ovary Syndrome Association of Australia
POSAA
PO Box 689
Kingswood
NSW 2747

(02) 8250 0222
www.posaa.asn.au
info@posaa.asn.au

ALTERNATIVE THERAPIES
Acupuncture Association of Victoria
1 Central Avenue
Moorabin
VIC 3189
03 9532 2480
Acupuncture Ethics and Standards Organization
275 Mogill Road
Indooroopilly QLD 4068
008 025 334
Australian Society of the Teachers of the Alexander Technique
19 Princess Street
Kew
VIC 3101
03 9853 1356
International Federation of Aromatherapists
1/390 Burwood Rd
Hawthorn
VIC 3122
03 9530 0067
National Herbalists Association of Australia
Suite 305
BST House
3 Smail Street
Broadway
New South Wales 2007
61 2 211 6437
Australian Institute of Homeopathy
21 Bulah Heights
Berdwra Heights
New South Wales 2082
Australian Federation of Homoeopaths
238 Ballarat Rd
Footscray
VIC 3011
03 9318 3057
The Australian Society of Clinical Hypnotherapists
200 Alexandra Parade
Fitzroy
VIC 3065
03 9418 3920

Association of Massage Therapists
18A Spit Road
Mosman
New South Wales
Australian Naturopathic Practitioners and Chiropractors Association
1st Floor, 609 Camberwell Road
Camberwell
VIC 3124
03 9889 0488
Naturopathic Physicians Association of Australia Inc
2 Beaumont Road
Canterbury
VIC 3126
03 9836 8103
Australian College of Nutritional and Environmental Medicine
13 Hilton Road
Beaumaris
VIC 3193
03 9589 6088
Australian Natural Therapists Association (ANTA)
PO Box 308
Melrose Park
South Australia
61-8-371-3222
Australian Association of Reflexology
2 Stewart Avenue
Matraville
NSW 2036
02 311 2322
Shiatsu Association of Australia
332 Carlisle Street
Balaclava
VIC 3183
03 9530 0067
BKS Iyengar Yoga Association of Australia Inc
Mosman
NSW
2 9969 4052
(freephone in Australia 1 800 677 037)
Endometriosis Association (Victoria) Inc
37 Andrew Crescent
South Croydon
VIC 3136
Tel 03 9870 0536
Fax 03 9870 3007

Index

daydreaming 125, 143
depression 128, 132, 150–2
detoxification 104–6
diabetes 71, 79, 87, 108, 154–7
diagnosis 2, 4–5, 7–8, 74–81
diet 45–9, 56–61, 98
   complementary therapies 93
   diabetes 156–7
   management 104, 106–9, 110–11
   stress 63–4, 65
   supplementation 166–7
   supplements 118
doctors 74–6, 82, 88, 95, 97, 100–1

eating disorders 65–7, 69, 128, 157–9
eggs 11, 17–19, 22–5, 31, 51
emotional help 126–45
endocrine disrupting chemicals
   (EDCs) 50–2
endometriosis 72
essential fatty acids (EFAs) 59–60,
   112
essential oils, see aromatherapy
exercise 61–3, 98, 111, 114, 125
   body image 129
   hirsutism 161
   irritability 177
   management plan 119–21
   period pain 184
   water 105

facial hair, see hirsutism
fainting 164–7
farming techniques 46–7
fat 53, 59–61, 107
fatigue 164–7

Fenton, David 171
fertility 13, 41, 70, 81, 91
   body image 127
   partnerships 138–9
   problems 96, 172–5
   self-esteem 133
   treatment 85–6
fertilization 19, 21, 24–5
follicle stimulating hormone (FSH)
   7, 20, 22–4, 29–31
   EDCs 52
   tests 79
   treatment 85–6
follicular phase 22–4
food
   cravings 167–70
   packaging 109
   processing 47, 55, 56, 70, 98
   pyramid 111, 112
   see also diet
forgiveness 128

genetics 12, 16, 18, 28
   causes 34, 38–40, 42–4
   diagnosis 80–1
   management 120
guilt 133

hair
   loss 29, 35, 170–1
   removal 161–4
   see also hirsutism 13–15
Hay, Louise 131
herbal teas 123
herbalism 92–4, 161
high blood pressure 70, 84, 108

PCOS Diet Book

How you can use the nutritional approach to deal with polycystic ovary syndrome

Colette Harris, With Theresa Cheung

The nutritional answer for all women sufferers of polycystic ovary syndrome – a condition which affects one in ten women

Having established herself as the authority on PCOS, Colette Harris now provides a practical plan for sufferers of Polycystic Ovary Syndrome with the *PCOS Diet Book*. The book explains how – with the right nutritional approach – you can lose weight, improve your skin, aid fertility and overcome exhaustion, depression and mood swings.

Various diets to suit each individual, accessible explanations of nutritional science and hormonal health, combined with an emphasis upon personal and emotional well-being make this title essential reading for all PCOS sufferers.

ISBN 0 00 7131844

Make
www.thorsonselement.com
your online sanctuary

Get online information, inspiration and guidance to help you on the path to physical and spiritual well-being. Drawing on the integrity and vision of our authors and titles, and with health advice, articles, astrology, tarot, a meditation zone, author interviews and events listings, www.thorsonselement.com is a great alternative to help create space and peace in our lives.

So if you've always wondered about practising yoga, following an allergy-free diet, using the tarot or getting a life coach, we can point you in the right direction.

www.thorsonselement.com • www.thorsonselement.com

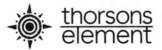
thorsons element